any time soon, as the concept of two or more species is a runaway train and many cannabis entrepreneurs are deeply invested in this sincere if misguided notion.

Because cannabis has been taken up diverse cultures over time, it has accrue Pot, hemp, bhang, goddess, ganja, weed boo, muggles, dope, charas, goddess, grass, viper, doob, pakololo, hash, hay, kif, and smoke are just a few of the myriad names by which cannabis is known. By any name, cannabis is one of the most widely employed mind- and mood-altering agents on Earth. In the United States approximately 52 percent of Americans over age eighteen have smoked marijuana. Though not as widely traded as coffee, nor as broadly consumed as alcohol, cannabis occupies a distinguished place in world agriculture and trade, as an agent of reverie and pleasure. Much of the trade history of cannabis has involved the use of low THC hemp for the making of hemp fiber, the most durable and environmentally sound fiber product on Earth. Hemp fiber makes superior rope, paper, clothing, and sailcloth. But it is the psychoactive cannabis, containing adequate amounts of THC, which concerns us here.

Penalties against possession of a drug should not be more damaging to an individual than the use of the drug itself.
PRESIDENT JIMMY CARTER

Legal tides for cannabis are finally changing, with legal medical and recreational cannabis in many U.S. states, with many more to follow. Draconian drug laws are rolling back in many parts of the world, and cannabis is the new dotcom boom. Major multinational beverage and tobacco companies have entered the cannabis market with billion-dollar investments, and some companies are making cannabinoids through yeast fermentation without any cannabis plants at all. It is getting wooly out there.

Despite a history of harsh penalties in many places for its possession, use, and sale, cannabis has been cultivated by millions of growers large and small, and it is shipped all over the planet. Hundreds of thousands of people have been thrown in prison for owning, purchasing, or selling this beneficial plant. This represents a huge injustice and a terribly ignorant policy. Cannabis has been carried on the backs of smugglers, poets, musicians, artists, lawmakers, government officials, soldiers, sailors, diplomats, actors, grandmothers, hippies, rednecks, truckers, laborers, explorers, botanists, attorneys, physicians, journalists, holy men, freethinkers, and buttoned-down business people. The allure of cannabis is so delightful and easily had; it is a sensuous magnet, a siren. Cannabis is not the property of one defined demographic type or another. Rather, it is a remarkable agent of reverie employed by all types, an equal opportunity mind-expander. This popularity demonstrates beautifully just how much people appreciate and value the effects of cannabis.

La cucaracha, la cucaracha	*The cockroach, the cockroach*
Ya no puede caminar	*Cannot walk anymore*
Porque no tiene	*Because it hasn't*
porque le falta	*because it lacks*
Marihuana que fumar	*marijuana to smoke*

CANNABIS, THE PLANT

Despite the best efforts of botanical experts to pinpoint the exact origin of cannabis, this information has proven elusive. But recent extensive sampling of pollen dating back millions of years may have identified the origin of this plant, which has provided food, fiber, medicine, and euphoria to humanity since the dawn of time. Attempting to settle the matter, researchers McPartland, Guy, and Hegman analyzed over five hundred pollen samples dating back to prehistoric times. The oldest cannabis pollen they discovered dated back to 19.6 million years ago in the Tibetan Plateau. The scientists conducting the study estimate that cannabis diverged from hops (*Humulus lupus*) around 28 million years ago. From the Tibetan Plateau cannabis reached Europe around 6 million years ago and China around 1.2 million years ago. The first cannabis pollen from India dates back 32,000 years.

An even more recent discovery has confirmed that humans employed cannabis for mind-expanding purposes. Wooden braziers found in the Jirzankal cemetery on the Pamir Plateau in western China date back 2,500 years and contain concentrated residues of cannabis rich in THC. The cannabis was likely smoked in mortuary ceremonies. According to Yimin Yang, a scientist at the University of Chinese Academy of Sciences, evidence suggests that cannabis was employed as an agent of spirit "to communicate with nature, or spirits, or deceased people."

Cannabis plants grow between one and twenty feet in height, with a furrowed central stalk from which numerous branches grow. The branches are covered with green leaves with long, green, toothed blades. There may be between three and fifteen blades per leaf, though the cannabis leaf is typically represented as having either five or seven blades. Virtually all parts of the cannabis plant above ground are covered with trichomes, fine hair-like growths covering most aerial (aboveground) plant tissues. Among the various types of trichomes, those known as capitate glandular trichomes contain a resin rich in cannabinoids, the phytochemicals that produce the distinctive psychoactive effects of this plant. Cannabis plants are either male or female, and the difference between the two becomes most apparent at the onset of flowering. Males flower prior to females and pollinate the females as they flower. Then the males begin to lose vigor and wither, while the females prosper and thrive.

Cannabis basically divides into two distinct types, psychoactive cannabis and hemp. This division occurred thousands of years ago, and both types have been part of human life since the end of the last ice age. The difference between the two is that hemp is nonpsychoactive and must by law contain less than 0.3 percent THC. In other words you cannot get high from hemp. Hemp yields seeds rich in healthy oil and protein, the stalks yield valuable and durable fiber, and the stalk, leaves, and buds of hemp yield CBD-rich oil, which is increasingly popular and broadly distributed. Psychoactive cannabis, typically called by its slang name marijuana, is our focus for the purposes of cannabis-infused yoga. I prefer the term *ganja*. Merlin and Clarke describe four morphological types of *Cannabis sativa*—narrow leaf drug (NLD), narrow leaf hemp (NLH), broad leaf drug (BLD), and broad leaf hemp (BLH).

The flowering buds and so-called sugar leaves of psychoactive cannabis plants NLD and BLD are used to smoke, eat, or make hashish, which is the concentrated resin. Flowers have a greater number of resin glands and are thus the most prized parts of the plant. Leaves of both male and female plants contain comparable levels of cannabinoids. But the flowers do not. In high-quality cannabis male flowers can produce a high. But in lower grades they may not do so at all. Female flowers, however, will be resinous and will produce a high. For this reason, growers apply their best agronomic efforts to increasing female bud size and yield, as well as potency. This is where the action resides. The techniques of cannabis cultivation are highly sophisticated at this point, and numerous highly potent hybrid varieties attest to the ingenuity of growers from British Columbia to California, to Jamaica, to Amsterdam, to Nepal.

In the keef dream the physical self was lulled into a state of unperturbed rest, while the higher mental faculties were stimulated to abnormal activity. The senses found Nirvana, the soul enfranchisement.

T. W. COAKLEY

Cannabis is an annual herb. During the warm season it grows from seeds obtained from female plants and then dies out. The plant grows in an astounding variety of soils and is decidedly not fussy, like coffee or cacao. Still, cannabis feeds heavily and takes a great deal of nutrients from the soil. The more fertile the soil, the better the quality of the cannabis. Cannabis maturation depends entirely on growing conditions and variety. Some hybrids can be grown to maturity under accelerated indoor cultivation in a scant two months. Others require as long as ten months to mature. Four or five months is typical.

Cannabis is generally hardy and disease resistant. However, young plants can be smothered by encroaching weeds, and cannabis plants in general can be damaged by wilt disease, leafspot disease, and branched broom rape. For the most part cannabis grows well in variable climate conditions and altitudes and variations in rainfall, care, and neglect. But heavy frosts will kill the plant.

Make the most you can of the Indian Hemp seed and sow it everywhere.

GEORGE WASHINGTON

To say that cannabis grows like a weed is no exaggeration. And though drug enforcement agencies around the world have attacked cannabis crops with alacrity, cultivation and yields continue to soar. In the United States corn belt, some farmers plant cannabis between corn rows. This keeps family farms from going under due to low commodity corn prices and results in massive tonnage of medium-quality weed. Nobody grows crops on a large scale like American farmers. Corn row cultivation represents a problem from a detection standpoint. Plots of cannabis are often located by aircraft using visual heat-sensing devices, as cannabis is a "hot" plant. It takes a lot of energy to grow, and it possesses a strong heat plume. But corn is an even hotter plant. When cannabis is cultivated between corn rows, visual methods of heat detection are rendered useless, as the heat plumes of the cannabis just disappear. But the greatest amount of high-quality U.S. grown cannabis comes out of California's Golden Triangle, Oregon, and Washington State, where so much fine ganja is cultivated that prices have cratered.

Cannabis is a major outdoor crop in California, Colorado, Oregon, Washington State, Hawaii, Mexico, Colombia, parts of the Andes, Jamaica, various Caribbean islands, and parts of Europe, Turkey, Morocco, Lebanon, Afghanistan, Southeast Asia, India, and Nepal. Its indoor cultivation, however, is occurring almost everywhere that electricity and water can be had. In the Netherlands indoor cultivation of cannabis is a multibillion-dollar enterprise. In British Columbia some of the world's most potent super-pot is cultivated almost entirely indoors. From Massachusetts to Madrid people cultivate a few plants or a few hundred plants in indoor growing areas where heat, light, moisture, and temperature can be controlled to produce maximum yields and potency. Growing chambers, lights, timers, and watering systems are available through various cannabis-related websites and publications and from garden stores.

CANNABIS, THE EUPHORIANT

Cannabis delivers an expansive, spacious high. For many, cannabis heightens sensory experience. It makes music more rich, food more tasty, colors more vivid, touch more sensual, sex more erotic. It also amplifies sensation and thus for our purposes here provides extra dimension to yoga practice. In some people cannabis stimulates creativity. In many, it provokes laughter.

The 1894 Indian Hemp Drugs Commission Report rather delightfully describes the effects of cannabis this way: "Bhang . . . makes the tongue of the lisper plain, freshens the intellect, and gives alertness to the body and gaiety to the mind. Such are the useful and needful ends for which the Almighty made bhang . . . Bhang is a cordial, a bile absorber, an appetizer, a prolonger of life. Bhang quickens fancy, deepens thought and braces judgement. . . . Bhang is the Joy-giver, the Sky-flier, the Heavenly guide, the poor man's Heaven, the soother of grief."

The enlivening, expansive, joy-producing effects of cannabis result from high-quality material employed judiciously. Consumed thoughtfully and in happy circumstances, cannabis increases pleasure and overall *joie de vivre*. Yet cannabis is so much more than a pleasure agent, as it also imparts a myriad of health benefits, with more benefits discovered every week. Cannabis provides relief for nausea, glaucoma, seizures, anxiety, depression, neurodegenerative disorders, and many more human health troubles. It is one of the great plant medicines, safe and versatile.

Everybody must get stoned.

BOB DYLAN

Cannabis produces its satisfying and euphoric effects thanks to THC, or D9-tetrahydrocannabinol, which is found in the resin glands produced on cannabis flowers and leaves of the female plant. Discovered in 1964 by Dr. Raphael Mechoulam and his colleagues at Israel's Weizmann Institute of Science, this compound is a member of a group of compounds known as the cannabinoids. Of these, over 110 are currently known. But it is mostly the THC content of cannabis alone that determines the potency of the material. THC and its broadly beneficial companion compound CBD, which is not psychoactive, occur in the greatest and second-greatest concentrations, respectively, of all the cannabinoids. In addition, more than 120 aromatic terpenes are produced on cannabis flowers and sugar leaves. These impart specific aromas to various cultivars of cannabis, including citrus and berry scents and skunky and woody ones. The terpenes also possess mood-modifying properties, enhancing alertness in some cases and plowing you into the couch in others. The many aromas of cannabis, from melon fragrances to berry, are all due to the varieties of aromatic terpenes. The main terpenes in cannabis are myrcene, limonene, linalool, caryophyllene, alpha-pinene and beta-pinene, alpha bisabolol, trans-nerolidol, humulene, delta-3-carene, camphene, borneol, terpineol, valencene, and geraniol. All of these compounds, the cannabinoids and the terpenes, occur on cannabis buds as hair-like crystals known as trichomes, similar in shape to tiny translucent mushrooms. It is this resinous material that, when vaporized, smoked, drunk, eaten, or otherwise consumed, delivers mind expansion.

When someone first smokes cannabis, and the conditions are right, something remarkable and concerning happens . . . The user is suddenly thrust upon a world of wonder, relaxation, humor, passion, creativity, and perhaps even gnosis.

STEPHEN GRAY

The discovery of the cannabinoids, specifically THC and CBD, has ushered in a whole new era of science and medicine. As I will describe, we have within us a relatively newly discovered master regulating system, the endocannabinoid system (ECS), which is fed perfectly by the cannabinoids in cannabis. The ECS exerts influence on almost all other body systems, from the cardiovascular system to the nervous system. Thus cannabinoids not only play a critical role in overall health, but, as I will elucidate, specifically enhance yoga practice as a result of feeding the ECS in a manner that stimulates energy and amplifies sensation.

THC activates specific ECS receptor sites in the brain, producing euphoria and relaxation. The acute toxicity of THC is extremely low, and in all of human history there has never been a single reported case of a death due to THC or cannabis consumption in any form. THC is lyophilic, and thus mixes well with various oils. For this reason, THC is readily dispersible in butter and other fats used in the making of cannabis baked goods and confections.

THC is rapidly absorbed and its various metabolites are eventually excreted in urine and feces. THC remains in tissues for a while and can still be detected in urine a couple of weeks after ingestion. THC has been isolated and purified into a prescription anti-emetic drug, Marinol (Dronabinol), which is available in 2.5, 5, and 10 milligram oral doses. But Marinol does not produce the same pleasures as whole cannabis consumption.

With cannabis all of the cannabinoids, along with the aromatic terpenes, act in concert to create effects more desirable and broader than the effects of a single purified molecule like THC. This "entourage effect," which is a way to describe synergy between multiple compounds, is argued persuasively by Dr. Ethan Russo, an ardent advocate of whole cannabis, and usually the smartest guy in whatever room he occupies. The same is true with whole green tea extract versus the purified green tea antioxidant EGCG, and with whole curcuminoid extract versus purified curcumin from turmeric. When you purify a single molecule from a plant, or synthesize a pure molecule originally found in a plant, the beneficial effects are reduced and the potentially unwanted effects are increased. This is almost universally so. Because there are so many variables possible with cannabis, growers worldwide are hard at work developing novel strains with signature aromas, flavors, and effects.

I'm a light user of marijuana. I see it as an elevator to shift my planes of consciousness. That's kind of the technical way I would say that I'm using it. I like to watch the way my mind works—in all the planes, and not in them at the same moment—on marijuana.

RAM DASS

Many excellent guides online can provide you with good information on the enlivening or sedative effects of different types of cannabis. I am a big fan of Himalayan-derived strains, finding them luminous, lively, and fragrant. But as they say in many product guides, your results may vary. Get recommendations on various strains, and perform bioassays. Your body-mind system is the most complex, marvelous, intricate, and sensitive of all analytical apparatus. Use your full senses to find out what you like, what works for you. Try them for yourself to ascertain your favorites. Figure out which cannabis strains and infusing methods are most helpful to your practice.

I began to gather the leaves of this plant and to eat them, and they have produced in me the gaiety that you witness. Come with me, then, that I may teach you to know it.

ANDREW KIMMENS, *TALES OF HASHISH*

As cannabis cultivation has become increasingly sophisticated, the concentration of THC has also increased, notably from the years after 1993, according to the *Journal of Forensic Sciences* in 2010. In the late 1960s we did in fact enjoy some perfectly potent cannabis, like Thai stick, Panama Red, Hawaiian Wowie, and Acapulco Gold. But sophisticated advances in cannabis cultivation have resulted in greater consistency of high-potency cannabis across the board, and even some with

THC values totaling a whopping 30 percent (though THC at around 15 to 20 percent or so is more typical and still very strong). The good side of this concentration is that a little bit goes a long way. For those who are going to smoke, this means burning and inhaling less material for the desired effect.

While cannabis may provoke hilarity or a keen appetite, it is rarely implicated in cases of violence and aggression. That is simply not the effect that cannabis imparts. Alcohol is clearly associated with the very worst forms of violent behavior and abuse, but cannabis is not. If anything, cannabis promotes a certain relaxed attitude. Cannabis tends to make people more mellow, disinclined to behave in an aggressive or violent manner. After consuming cannabis users would rather hang with friends and enjoy themselves than go out and beat up somebody.

Much of the prevailing public apprehension about marijuana may stem from the drug's effect of inducing introspection and bodily passivity, which are antipathetic to a culture that values aggressiveness, achievement, and activity.

THE NEW COLUMBIA ENCYCLOPEDIA

I disagree with the previous "bodily passivity" characterization of effects from the *Columbia Encyclopedia*. Some people can and do sink into the couch and become fixed there, thus the term *couch lock*. This effect can be the result of a concentration of sedative terpenes in a particular strain. But equally many people consume cannabis before performing various types of work, rather than dissolving into a cushion. I stack wood for our home woodstove and typically light up before doing so. It makes the very repetitive task more pleasurable, more of a flow. In fact cannabis can be terrific for engaging in long hours of physical labor.

Opinions of cannabis and its effects are highly polarized. Some people regard cannabis use as a menace, an evil that destroys the mind and corrupts the very fabric of society. Fortunately this position is dissolving in the face of reality. Others regard cannabis use as a fairly innocuous and pleasant pastime, which should be completely legalized without further ado. Despite this apparent gulf one thing is certain: Cannabis is with us to stay. Its use continues to spread. Drug eradication efforts have only inspired more cleverness and caution on the part of growers, dealers, and users. Cannabis is now being more thoughtfully considered by a greater number of people than ever before in history. Cannabis plays an important role in the ongoing human inclination to modify mind and mood, and it will not go away. The irrepressible power of enjoyment is a crushing opponent of fear and misinformation.

The actual experience of the smoked herb has been clouded by a fog of dirty language perpetrated by a crowd of fakers who have not had the experience and yet insist on downgrading it.

ALLEN GINSBERG

CANNABIS TRAVELS

Cannabis has most likely been a companion of humans since the advent of agriculture, around ten thousand years ago. Cannabis has been cultivated for its fiber, its oil, its nutritious seeds, and its psychoactive buds. Hemp fibers six thousand years old have been found in China. The emperor and revered herbalist Shen Nung wrote about cannabis in 2000 BCE, recommending its use for rheumatic pain, constipation, and female disorders. The emperor commented that cannabis "makes one communicate with spirits and lightens one's body." In early China cannabis was used in magical ceremonies for divination. Later, around 200 CE, the herbalist and surgeon Hua Tuo employed cannabis in wine as an anesthetic.

In India cannabis fit well into the traditional folk medicine. The plant was referred to in the ancient *Artha Veda,* which may have been written as early as the treatise by Shen Nung. The plant was recommended for a variety of health needs, from relieving dysentery to improving digestion, easing headache to improving judgment. The *Rajanirghanta,* penned around 300 CE, recommended cannabis to alleviate flatulence, stimulate appetite, and boost memory. The later *Tajni Guntu* described cannabis as a strengthener, a promoter of success, a mover of laughter, and a sexual excitant. In the Hindu tantras cannabis is described as an empowering intoxicant. The plant was made into "pills of gaiety." Its psychoactive properties gave cannabis high status as a divine elixir, a life-promoting, soul-vitalizing agent. In the Indian Himalayas and the Tibetan Plateau, cannabis achieved high religious esteem.

Like other beloved psychoactive plants, cannabis traveled far and wide, carried by pilgrims, traders, and sailors. Known as a camp follower, cannabis spread as its seeds were dispersed where it was consumed, following people on trade routes and other passages. One historical account states that in ancient times an Indian pilgrim introduced cannabis use to Khorasan (northeastern Iran). From there cannabis spread to Chaldea (the southernmost valley of the Tigris and Euphrates Rivers), then into Syria, Egypt, and Turkey. Hair analysis of Egyptian mummies dated back to 1070 BCE reveals high levels of cannabis residues. This puts the spread of cannabis into Egypt prior to that time. Early Arabian manuscripts describe the Garden of Cafour near Cairo as a major location for the use of hashish by fakirs.

Sometime around 450 BCE the Greek historian Herodotus recounted the use of cannabis by Scythian horsemen in central Asia. The Greek writer said, "they make a booth by fixing in the ground three sticks inclined towards one another, and stretching around them woolen felts, which they arrange so as to fit as close as possible: inside the booth a dish is placed upon the ground, into which they put a number of red hot stones and then add some hemp seed. . . . The Scythians, as I said, take some of this hemp-seed, and, creeping under the felt coverings, throw it upon the red-hot stones; immediately it smokes and gives out such a vapor as no Grecian vapor bath can exceed: the Scyths, delighted, shout for joy . . ."

By God, bravo, hashish! It stirs deep meanings. Don't pay attention to those who blame it. Refrain from the daughter of the vines. And do not be stingy with it. Eat it dry always and live! By God, Bravo, hashish!

It is above pure wine. When noble men use it, eat and agree, young man. Eating it revives the dead. By God, Bravo, hashish!

It gives the stupid, inexperienced, dull person the cleverness of a straightforward sage. I don't think I can escape from it.

By God, bravo, hashish!

FROM A THIRTEENTH-CENTURY ARABIAN TALE

The account given by Herodotus has been confirmed in archaeological digs, with the discovery of apparatus as described. However, residues show that cannabis bracts, leaves, and buds rich with cannabinoids and terpenes were the materials that produced Scythian euphoria, not just the seeds. The Scythians took cannabis, their joygiver, across Asia westward to Europe. An urn found in Berlin and dated around 500 BCE contained cannabis leaves and seeds. Within a short period cannabis had made its way to England, Scotland, and Ireland.

Archaeological evidence shows that the Assyrians used cannabis for incense during the first millennium BCE. Hashish especially became popular, spreading throughout Asia Minor during the first millennium CE, and from there into Africa. Tribespeople in Africa, notably the Bushmen, Kaffirs, and Hottentots (who called cannabis *dacha*), embraced the euphoria-producing effects of cannabis. The plant and its use were taken up enthusiastically throughout Africa.

In the thirteenth century Marco Polo recounted the exciting tale of the Hashishan, or Assassins, a group of Nizari Ismailis who were followers of a mysterious "Old Man of the Mountain." According to history the warlord Hasan ibn al-Sabah resided in the mountain fortress of

Alamut, south of the Caspian Sea. Hasan ibn al-Sabah reputedly intoxicated young recruits with hashish and indulged them with women and all manner of pleasures. Informing the soldiers that such rewards would be theirs as a result of unwavering service to him, he garnered extreme loyalty among his troops. The young Hashishan were bold, fierce, fearless, and willing to sacrifice themselves for their leader's cause, assured of a hash-intoxicated, sex-rich idyllic afterlife. The Assassins spread throughout Persia and Syria, becoming a much-feared sect. It's a fascinating tale, yet completely apocryphal. Marco Polo recounted a fabulous, if untrue, yarn. The Assassins were real, but there is no evidence to support the notion that they were promised entrance into the kingdom of heaven via an infusion of hashish. Still, it's fun to imagine a band of sword-wielding assassins howling down out of the Persian hills, fire in their hearts and hashish in their brains.

Cannabis may even have been mentioned as *pannag* in the Bible, in Ezekiel 27:17. Pannag is linguistically similar to the Sanskrit bhang. Are the visions of Ezekiel the psychedelic results of cannabis consumption? In Jerusalem remains of burned cannabis show its use there around 400 CE. In Exodus 30:22–23, fragrant cane is believed to be *kaneh bosm,* cannabis. This makes sense. *Cannabis* means "cane-like." And while sugar cane has no discernable aroma of significance, budding cannabis, or fragrant cane, certainly does. Fresh ripe buds of cannabis are profuse with terpenes. Fragrant cane was part of a biblical recipe for holy anointing oil.

In 200 CE Greek physician and philosopher Galen wrote that hemp was sometimes given to guests for their enjoyment. In 77 CE Pliny the Elder mentioned cannabis in his *Naturalis Historia.* But cannabis became an item of value in early Europe primarily for its fiber. Merry Olde England took up cannabis with vigor, and during the Anglo Saxon period from 400–1100 CE, the plant was produced on a large scale for its fiber. The superiority of hemp fiber for maritime purposes ensured not only that cannabis would sail the seas among the seafaring explorers and traders of Europe, but that its cultivation would spread far and wide as well.

In 1378 the Arabian Emir Soudoun Sheikouni placed a ban on the use of cannabis and imposed penalties and imprisonment for its use. Despite this, cannabis use flourished unabated. This is the first known ban on cannabis, which would be repeatedly insulted in this manner throughout history.

The historical record shows that Spanish sailors introduced cannabis to Chile in 1545 and to Peru in 1554. However, analysis of Peruvian mummies dated from 200–1500 CE shows traces of cannabis. This suggests earlier contact between the Americas and Asia or Egypt. African slaves who arrived in South America in the seventeenth and eighteenth centuries contributed to the spread of cannabis in that region. In many parts of Africa cannabis was already well established and widely used.

In the 1840s French doctor Jacques Joseph Moreau published several papers on the use of cannabis for mental illness. His 1945 publication *Hashish and Mental Illness: Psychological Studies* became famous and sparked great interest in the use of cannabis and its concentrated resin. In 1846 Moreau and Theophile Gauthier established *Le Club des Hashischins* (the hashish users' club). With its exotic drug and Arabian theme, the club became a hot spot for writers including Alexandre Dumas, Honoré de Balzac, Charles Baudelaire, and numerous others. This concrescence of hashish and the literati sparked a profusion of literary accounts of cannabis use and greatly popularized the plant and its use among the cognoscenti. Hoisted high on the shoulders of some of the greatest literary figures of that time, cannabis became an exotic cause célèbre.

British sailors dutifully delivered cannabis to Canada in 1606 and to Virginia in 1611. In 1632 the Pilgrims brought cannabis to New England. But the low resin cannabis was used for hemp fiber, not for euphoria. While hemp was made into rope in the north, south of the border, things were a bit different. Cannabis was used for psychoactive purposes by the Tepecano Indians of northwest Mexico, and migrant Mexican laborers introduced marijuana smoking to the southwestern United States. These laborers, as well as African slaves, established cannabis use in the South. From its agricultural roots in the Southwest and Deep South, cannabis smoking spread to the jazz world in New Orleans, and from there to numerous cities in the United States.

I found the drug well known to the negroes of the Southern United States and of Brazil, although few of their owners had ever heard of it.

EXPLORER SIR RICHARD FRANCIS BURTON, 1885

In 1893 the British government, concerned over widespread cannabis use in its colony of India, commissioned the now famous 3,200-page, seven-volume Indian Hemp Commission Report. This extensive survey detailed the history and use of cannabis throughout the Indian subcontinent and its people. The report concluded that cannabis use was of little concern to health, and that "[m]oderate use of hemp drugs produces no injurious effects on the mind . . ."

From 1860–1900 the Gunjah Wallah Company made Gunjah Wallah Hasheesh Candy, which was distributed throughout the United States by druggists. Highly successful, the maple-flavored electuary was sold as the Gunjah Of Enchantment and was advertised in this way: "TRUE SECRET OF YOUTH AND BEAUTY. It is a remedy that ought to be in every house on account of its harmlessness and potency. And above all, because of its exceeding cheapness. It is the cheapest remedy in the world. Colds readily yield to it."

Gunjah Wallah had its enthusiasts, though few as highly visible as General Robert E. Lee of the Confederacy, who said, "I wish it was in my power to place a Dollar Box of the HASHEESH CANDY into the pocket of every Confederate Soldier, because I am convinced that it speedily relieves Debility, Fatigue, and Suffering."

Drug giant Parke Davis was also a major player in the cannabis medicine market with its fluid extract of Cannabis Americana.

Intense anti-cannabis crusading in the United States in the 1930s made the plant illegal to possess and use in August 1937. America's first drug czar, Henry Anslinger, went on a rampage against cannabis, ratcheting up his battle cries against the plant until its eventual prohibition. DuPont chemical company, who wished to protect the market for petroleum-derived plastic against the encroachment of superior cannabis-derived plastic, fought alongside the Hearst newspaper group, whose extensive forest and pulp holdings were potentially threatened by superior hemp paper. Using the Hearst papers as a mouthpiece for baseless propaganda describing "marijuana" as a destroyer of youth and a promoter of insanity, Anslinger and large anti-cannabis corporate interests lied to and deceived legislators and the public about what had previously been known as an innocuous plant with medical value. Implicit in their utterly dishonest accounts was the notion that brown-skinned men were employing cannabis to turn innocent white women into sex slaves. This racist phobia sealed the deal for prohibition. Yet despite onerous legal penalties, cannabis use continued to expand. In the 1950s marijuana smoking was embraced by members of the Beat movement and writers of that time, including Jack Kerouac, Allen Ginsberg, Alice Toklas, William S. Burroughs, and other influential literary figures.

Euphoria and brilliant storms of laughter; ecstatic reveries and extension of one's personality on several simultaneous planes are to be complacently expected. Almost anything Saint Theresa did, you can do better.

ALICE B. TOKLAS, REFERRING TO THE EFFECTS OF THE LEGENDARY HASCHICH FUDGE RECIPE IN HER *THE ALICE B. TOKLAS COOK BOOK* PUBLISHED IN 1954. THE RECIPE FOR THE PSYCHOACTIVE FUDGE WAS SUPPLIED BY BRION GYSIN, AN ARTIST LIVING IN TANGIER MOROCCO.

With my inexhaustible supply of Elitch (cannabis), I daily dive into these dim regions and crawl to the surface with the stub of a pencil, sweating, to record what I have observed.

JACK KEROUAC

In the 1960s marijuana became the burning emblem of a new generation and the hippie era. Pot smoking spread across the United States, as millions turned on with cannabis and psychedelic rock music. American poet and author of *Howl* Allen Ginsberg openly promoted the pleasurable uses of cannabis in the 1960s and was famously photographed wearing a sandwich sign that read "Pot Is Fun." That explosion reverberated throughout the world. Since the 1960s cannabis has become increasingly popular worldwide. The growth of the Rastafarian movement in Jamaica not only further popularized cannabis, but helped to produce reggae, a vastly popular, ganja-inspired musical genre. Bob Marley, Peter Tosh, and other Rastafarian entertainers smoked cannabis openly on stage at performances, flying their freak flags high and in plain sight. Woodstock in August 1969 is likely the largest cannabis smoke-in in history to this day, featuring three days of peace, love, rock and roll, and lots of mind-altering substances.

The Indians get no usefulness from this, unless it is the fact that they become ravished by ecstasy, and delivered from all worries and cares, and laugh at the least little thing.

GARCIA DA ORTA, 1563

Today a majority of U.S. states have medical or recreational cannabis laws, with more on the way. Cannabis products, including oils, waxes, vapes, flower, and edibles, now fill "dispensary" shelves. A cannabis green rush is fully underway. Cannabis edibles are a big emerging category, and cannabis cookery is a popular and emerging dimension of culinary art. Cannabis will take a big bite out of the market for benzodiazepine anxiety drugs, SSRIs, sleep drugs, and more. This will cause long overdue and well-deserved financial chaos in the pharmaceutical industry. Cannabis is currently being employed in psychotherapy to assist some clients to relax and open up more candidly, with good results. And experiential churches, from the Abrahamic religion Rastafari to modern

Elevationists, are employing cannabis as a sacrament in services.

Since its first use by humans thousands of years ago, cannabis has proven an unstoppable force. Eradication efforts have failed miserably, as they run counter to the natural human tendency to seek satisfying pleasure through friendly plants. Today cannabis is employed by hundreds of millions of people. Times have changed and continue to change, and a more sane attitude toward cannabis prevails.

Fragrant smoke from the Arabian plant's brown juice creates a swirling dance of powerful fantasies.
MORITZ VON SCHWIND

CANNABIS AS MEDICINE

Cannabis has been employed as a valuable medicine since antiquity. Today the medical marijuana movement is steadily gathering steam, even as some lawmakers are cautious about their reelection if they follow suit. Since 1996 thirty-three states and the District of Columbia have legalized cannabis to some extent or another. Eleven states have legalized recreational cannabis, allowing for personal use, transport, and cultivation of this beneficial and safe plant medicine.

Though the U.S. government denies any known medical value of whole cannabis, this is just sleight of mouth. In fact, the federal government has run a medical marijuana program out of the University of Mississippi since 1978. Called the Compassionate Investigational New Drug program or Compassionate IND and administered by the National Institutes of Drug Abuse, the program provides cannabis joints in large cans on a monthly basis to a limited number of people who qualify for the program. Each can contains three hundred pre-rolled joints of cannabis grown, dried, and prepared by this federal program at Ole Miss. Today Compassionate IND is on the wane with only four remaining patients, and no new patients accepted into the program. Go Feds.

Cannabis is the single most versatile herbal remedy, and the most useful plant on Earth. No other single plant contains as wide a range of medically active herbal constituents.
ETHAN RUSSO, M.D.

In poll after poll a majority of Americans support the medical use of marijuana. At this point hundreds of medical organizations, educational centers, nurse associations, and other health bodies support greater access to cannabis medicine. The full legalization of cannabis for personal medical use would alleviate a lot of suffering.

If it is perceived that the Public Health Service is going around and giving marijuana to folks, there would be a perception that this stuff can't be so bad. It gives a bad signal.
JAMES MASON, M.D., FORMER HHS ASSISTANT
SECRETARY FOR HEALTH AND HEAD OF
THE U.S. PUBLIC HEALTH SERVICE

In traditional systems of medicine such as India's Ayurveda, cannabis has enjoyed millennia of use as a valuable medicine. Cannabis is recommended for relief of pain and headaches, for increasing appetite, for promoting sleep in cases of insomnia, for subduing hysteria, and for easing painful menstruation. Until 1941 marijuana was listed in the U.S. Pharmacopoeia as an approved drug. Today cannabis is listed as a Schedule I drug, on a par with crack and heroin. This designation is not only fundamentally unfair, but is incorrect. Cannabis is not a narcotic, and it shows great benefits as a medicine. But the conversation about medical cannabis is intensifying as research from around the globe demonstrates significant benefits. Medical cannabis research focuses primarily on the efficacy of cannabis in analgesia, relieving nausea and vomiting, counteracting wasting syndrome by means of appetite stimulation, and inhibiting the progress of glaucoma. In each of these areas cannabis demonstrates real and significant value. In this cause Israel is a science leader. U.S. drug authorities prohibit studies of cannabis except those designed to show harm, whereas Israel supports good science wherever it may lead. At present the United States is left way behind in the careful study of the most widely beneficial plant on Earth, due to inept politics.

The two primary types of *Cannabis sativa,* psychoactive cannabis— let's use the term *ganja*—and hemp, yield different compounds in different concentrations. Ganja is rich in THC, the most abundant of all the cannabinoids. Known for promoting a high, THC relieves pain and is widely employed for this purpose. For many, THC promotes relaxation and greater ease. Ganja typically heightens the sense of sight, hearing, smell, touch, and taste. It also significantly enhances sexual pleasure, a use for which it is very widely employed. For some, ganja is a stimulant. I find that I can apply myself to hard or repetitive tasks with greater ease with ganja. But many people find that ganja aids sleep. And since so many people suffer from inadequate sleep, this is a sought-after effect. A famous effect of ganja for some is the munchies. Many people crave snacks when they consume ganja. This makes it helpful for chemotherapy sufferers. Chemotherapy most often kills appetite, but ganja can help to restore that. Additionally ganja promotes peace and reduces aggression. There are good reasons that so many people turn to cannabis as medicine, especially psychoactive ganja.

In the burgeoning cannabis market, CBD products derived from hemp have soared in popularity. Cultivation of non-psychoactive hemp is legal nationwide and CBD supplements are now the most popular herbal supplements in the United States. And while CBD products lag behind ganja in the market, the rush is definitely on, with everything infused with CBD, from beverages to gummies to tinctures to vapes. CBD also relieves pain, and it is a first-rate anti-inflammatory. Pain is virtually epidemic, and CBD provides real relief. Many people turn to CBD-based products for joint pain and to relieve pain from injuries. For mild to moderate anxiety, CBD-based products help greatly in many cases, and make a safer and preferred alternative to the benzo-diazepine class of drugs, which includes Valium, Xanax, Serax, Ativan, and Klonopin. CBD demonstrates blood-sugar-regulating properties and is of value in relieving nausea. For children with seizure conditions, CBD can help to significantly reduce the total number and severity of seizures. CBD is somewhat antidepressant as well. CBD-based products help makers to avoid running afoul of narcotics laws, and thus CBD products are only increasing in popularity.

In a review of sixty articles, a paper in *Clinical Psychology Review* in 2017 detailed the beneficial use of cannabis for treating PTSD and substance abuse disorders, notably addiction to opioids. Not only is cannabis not the much-feared "gateway drug" that critics deride, but it can actually be of medicinal value in the fight against addiction to dangerous and potentially lethal opioids, including a host of toxic prescription drugs. The same paper found benefits for depression and social anxiety.

Analgesia

Pain is one of the most common conditions for which drug treatment is sought. Pain comes in varied forms. Neuropathic pain is caused by damage or abnormality anywhere along a nerve. Nociceptive pain origi-nates as a result of inflammation around an injury. The two types can occur at the same time, depending on the nature of physical damage. Postsurgical pain is very common, affecting almost everybody who undergoes any kind of surgical procedure. Cancer pain is caused by tumor growth into sensitive areas, and by cancer surgery and radiation. Whatever the cause, pain can range from mild to completely debilitat-ing. Any agent that can help is valuable.

In almost all painful maladies I have found Indian Hemp by far the most useful of drugs.

J. RUSSELL REYNOLDS, M.D.,
PHYSICIAN TO QUEEN VICTORIA

Cannabis is an excellent, time-tested analgesic. This was first brought to light to Westerners by Dr. W. B. O'Shaughnessy in the 1840s. O'Shaughnessy studied the uses of cannabis for pain in Indian traditional medicine and conducted both animal and human experiments for this purpose. In the nineteenth century tincture of cannabis was commonly used as an analgesic. Since the mid-1800s hundreds of articles on the analgesic uses of cannabis appeared in British and American journals.

The cannabinoids appear to be both central nervous system (CNS) pain depressants and anti-inflammatory pain relievers. The mechanisms for these activities are complex. While THC is the primary cannabinoid studied, others including cannabidiol and hexahydrocannabinol have also been the subjects of research. When all results are eventually tallied, I do not doubt that whole cannabis resin, rich in THC, will prove superior for pain relief than any single isolated agent.

In animal studies THC produces decreased sensitivity to pain and reduced inflammation in a variety of tests. In live, hurting human beings, THC reduces pain in cases of cancer. Nabilone, a synthetic version of THC (Eli Lilly), has demonstrated relief of pain in cases of multiple sclerosis, spinal injury, peripheral neuropathy, and malignancy. But nabilone is just a path for a pharmaceutical company to cash in on cannabis. A full-spectrum THC and CBD-rich flower extract will not only function similarly from a benefit standpoint, but the entourage effect of all the support compounds in the extract make it superior in efficacy and overall health value. Plus, nabilone offers a host of potentially nasty negative effects, and whole cannabis extract offers few. As the cannabis market explodes with multibillion-dollar products and campaigns, remember that the whole plant and its full-spectrum extracts, not isolated molecules, are the real deal for health and healing.

By far the greatest number of people who find pain relief in cannabis either smoke or eat the drug and its preparations. Entities such as the Oakland Cannabis Buyers' Cooperative and the San Francisco Cannabis Buyers' Club have dispensed medical marijuana to numerous people, including those in pain, for decades. Reports from the field far exceed in volume the results yielded by small, clinical tests.

Cannabis relieves pain. For suffering humanity this is a good and valuable thing.

Nausea and Wasting Syndrome

There's nothing like a toxic dose of chemotherapy to put you on your knees, clutching the rim of the toilet, head in the bowl, puking your guts out. Chemotherapy makes all your hair fall out, causes tremendous nausea and vomiting, kills appetite, causes serious wasting, and puts people in the grave. Plus, it costs a fortune. And it's legal. Cannabis makes people feel good, does none of the above, and kills nobody. It's illegal in many places, and in some countries and states you can still be thrown in prison for its use.

As far as mitigating nausea and stemming vomiting caused by chemotherapy is concerned, the jury is back on cannabis. In whole cannabis form or as nabilone, the cannabinoids have been shown in several dozen human studies to reduce nausea and vomiting in patients suffering from chemotherapy poisoning. The cannabinoids perform as well as or better than other prescription drugs for the same purpose. Some studies show—no surprise—that smoked cannabis works better than orally ingested THC pills. This route of ingestion is quicker in action and produces a superior nausea-quelling effect. There is no question whatsoever that cannabis reduces vomiting in chemotherapy sufferers.

Another effect of chemotherapy, and a typical effect of AIDS, is wasting due to loss of appetite. For this condition cannabis is a tremendous boon, promoting appetite in individuals who otherwise have no desire to eat. In studies of chemotherapy sufferers, cannabis improved appetite. Countless AIDS patients have used cannabis for the same purpose, with good results. For patients suffering from chemotherapy poisoning or AIDS, cannabis improves appetite, prevents weight loss, and improves mood. What compassionate human being on this Earth would deny cannabis to these people?

Glaucoma

The most common cause of blindness in the Western world, glaucoma is characterized by increased intraocular pressure. This pressure is caused by a blockage in the channels that regulate the eye's internal fluid. An even balance of fluid maintains the healthy spherical shape of the eye. But increased fluid and pressure can damage the optic nerve, resulting in blindness. In both animals and humans, smoking or eating cannabis results in reduced intraocular pressure. A few studies and numerous anecdotal reports indicate that cannabis can play a valuable role in stemming the progress of glaucoma.

Epileptic Seizures

A few studies point to anti-epileptic activity with cannabis, notably with CBD-rich preparations. A 2016 article in *Lancet* investigated the effects of CBD on patients aged one to thirty with treatment-resistant severe epilepsy, and found that "cannabidiol might reduce seizure frequency and might have an adequate safety profile in children and young adults with highly treatment-resistant epilepsy." Today the CBD drug Epidiolex is approved in the United States to treat treatment-resistant severe epilepsy. This is another pharma offering, a highly purified CBD product derived from cannabis. A CBD-rich hemp oil offers a more wholesome, nutritious, and effective option.

Antioxidant

In October of 2003 our own United States government filed a patent entitled "Cannabinoids as Antioxidants and Neuroprotectants" making the case that "[c]annabinoids have been found to have antioxidant properties, unrelated to NMDA receptor antagonism. This new-found property makes cannabinoids useful in the treatment and prophylaxis of a wide variety of oxidation associated diseases, such as ischemic, age-related, inflammatory, and autoimmune diseases. The cannabinoids are found to have particular application as neuroprotectants, for example in limiting neurological damage following ischemic insults, such as stroke and trauma, or in the treatment of neurodegenerative diseases, such as Alzheimer's disease, Parkinson's disease, and HIV dementia."

The government can't just get a patent because they think it's a good idea. They have to demonstrate that there is validity to any claims made for such a patent. To support the potential use of cannabinoids for inflammatory and auto-immune disorders, Alzheimer's, Parkinson's, and more, they backed up their patent with high-quality scientific references. The patent was filed so that the government could profit by assigning rights to different companies and garnering royalties for cannabinoid-based drugs they might develop for the above purposes. Canny U.S. officials, certain that cannabis would be a multibillion-dollar industry, set themselves up to profit from the great cannabis green rush.

Alzheimer's Disease

Apropos of the government's cannabis patent, there is some intriguing science around cannabis and Alzheimer's. A study published in *Molecular Pharmaceutics* reported that THC reduced the formation of amyloid plaque in the brain, which is associated with the progression of the disease. Amyloid plaque is not presumed to cause Alzheimer's, but it does co-occur and increase as symptoms progress. The inhibition of plaque and its elimination are considered valuable to overall brain health.

Anxiety

In 2017 researchers at the University of Illinois and the University of Chicago reported that low level intake of THC helped to quell anxiety, while higher doses tended to exacerbate anxiety. This was the conclusion of a study of forty-two volunteers aged eighteen to forty. Psychiatrist Emma Childs, who supervised the study, commented, "Our findings provide some support for the common claim that cannabis is used to reduce stress and relieve tension and anxiety. At the same time, our finding that participants in the higher THC group reported small but significant increases in anxiety and negative mood throughout the test supports the idea that THC can also produce the opposite effect."

The biggest killer on the planet is stress, and I still think the best medicine is and always has been cannabis.

WILLIE NELSON

Multiple Sclerosis

A study in the *Canadian Medical Association Journal* reported on thirty MS patients with treatment-resistant muscle spasticity. In patients who smoked cannabis, spasticity dropped by about 30 percent, while there was no drop among those in the placebo group. Today the full-spectrum cannabis drug Sativex is approved among twenty-five countries including the UK, Canada, Spain, and New Zealand to treat MS-related spasticity.

Other Healing Experiences

Though some people accept only double-blind, placebo-controlled crossover clinical trials as evidence of medicinal efficacy, others accept real-life human experience as valid for sorting out what works and what doesn't. Too many reports to ignore indicate that cannabis can provide valuable relief in cases of menstrual cramps, hypertension, anxiety, muscle spasms, epilepsy, asthma, rheumatic pain, and anxiety. Without question cannabis offers real help to many people who suffer from various health disorders. Cannabis is in many cases as effective as other medications. In many instances it is far safer. Medical use is not the primary use of cannabis worldwide. But for those who turn to cannabis for relief, it is good medicine indeed.

CANNABIS PLANT SPIRIT

Everything that exists possesses a unique energetic signature, by virtue of its composition, weight, size, and other characteristics. The unique energetic signature of living entities of all types represents the spirit of that thing. Spirit is essence, the fundamental and primary nature. Plants all have spirits, and it is possible to commune with plants in such a way as to garner knowledge and to harness healing power. I have spent decades with shamans, most notably in the Amazon and the Andes, where communing with and harnessing the healing power of plants is a common approach to healing practices.

Cannabis is not only a very popular plant much beloved and broad in healing power, but it is what is known as a master plant, one imbued with high energy, and extremely powerful in nature. The master plants are employed by shamans and various healers to assist in healing and divination by harnessing not just the phytochemical properties of those plants, but their immense spirits as well. These are plant allies. They help healers and seers to harness the forces of nature in various ways.

This may all sound like fantasy. Especially if you were raised in an urban or otherwise de-natured environment, communing with plant spirits may be utterly unfamiliar and seemingly fictitious. I do understand. But I will tell you that you lose nothing and may gain much by giving the spirit of cannabis real consideration. Even if this seems like a mere act of imagination, give it a try for a time. Especially after infusing, tend your mind toward the spirit of cannabis with focused intent, requesting access to the immense healing and divinatory power of the plant.

Do not imagine that you are communing with a person. A plant is not likely to strike up a conversation. But by connecting with this plant via a quiet, energized, and focused mind, you can gain access to the intelligent vastness of cannabis spirit. My own forays deep into that have assured me that cannabis is one of the most powerful and most beneficial of all plant allies on Earth. An ally assists. In the case of cannabis-infused yoga, the spirit of cannabis opens you, allows more energetic inflow, expands your capacity to delve deeply into sense and sensation, and into the ocean of energy within you.

We do not see radio waves passing through the air, TV signals traveling across vast space, or satellite signals bouncing around the Earth or Wi-Fi frequency bands. Yet we know these various emissions and frequencies are real by how we receive them. So, too, you can know the spirit of cannabis by how you receive it. The big difference is that you are using the sophisticated instrumentation of your body and mind, not a box with dials and an electric plug. You possess vast power in your cells, many millions of volts worth. And cannabis has a massive charge as well. By linking your consciousness and your focused intent with the spirit of cannabis, you gain an ally of imponderable power.

MEET YOUR ECS

Even though humans have delved deeply into the anatomy, physiology, and functions of the body for as long as we have existed, we are still learning new things to this day. The mapping of the human genome and its workings and our understanding of the microbiome are relatively new, and have given us far greater options for promoting health. So, too, the discovery of the ECS—the endocannabinoid system—has revolutionized our understanding of some of the very basics of human health across many body systems. It seems inconceivable that we did not know about the ECS sooner, as it is a master regulating system that exerts great influence over the most vital aspects of human health and well-being.

As I mentioned previously THC was discovered in 1964 by Dr. Raphael Mechoulam and his colleagues at Israel's Weizmann Institute of Science. Widely considered the godfather of cannabinoid science, Dr. Mechoulam and his many brilliant collaborators have continued to this day to plumb the remarkable world of the ECS and the various cannabinoids that in some way or another affect its function. Since the discovery of THC many other brilliant scientists have also made key advances in this field.

In 1998, while conducting a study at St. Louis University School of Medicine, professor of physiology Dr. Allyn Howlett and pharmacologist Dr. William Devane determined that the brains of mammals possess receptor sites that react to cannabinoids. These sites, dubbed cannabinoid receptors, turn out to be the most abundant neurotransmitter receptor sites in the brain. In 1990 Dr. Lisa Matsuda at the National Institutes of Health cloned this receptor, which is known as CB1. This allowed scientists to determine the effects of exposing the CB1 receptor to various substances. At about the same time, the CB2 receptor was discovered and subsequently cloned. The CB1 and CB2 receptors are broadly distributed throughout the central and peripheral nervous systems. In the brain these receptors are located in the brain stem, cerebral cortex, hippocampus, cerebellum, basal ganglia, hypothalamus, and amygdala. They are also found in the liver, kidneys, spleen, gonads, and heart.

Shortly after the discovery of the CB2 receptor, two graduate Ph.D. students of Raphael Mechoulam, Dr. Lumir Hanus and Dr. William Devane, and their team at Hebrew University in Jerusalem discovered anandamide (AEA), an endogenous (made in the body) cannabinoid. *Ananda* is the Sanskrit word for "bliss," and is used to describe yogic ecstasy. It is a perfect name for the compound, as anandamide is equal to THC in psychoactivity. In other words we make in our own bodies a compound that by its very nature and by our basic biology promotes mind expansion. Chocolate also contains anandamide, which may attribute to the cacao plant's botanical name *Theobroma cacao,* food of the gods. Black truffles, too, contain anandamide. Subsequent to the discovery of anandamide, the same doctors and their team discovered another major endocannabinoid, 2-arachidonoylglycerol (2-AG), along with several others.

———

We decided to name the new brain-derived ligand anandamide. Bill (Devane) was learning Sanskrit at the time and suggested "Ananda" (supreme joy in this ancient tongue).

RAPHAEL MECHOULAM, PH.D.

———

As scientists explored the receptors CB1 and CB2, and as they worked to understand the various cannabinoids and the pathways by which these agents work, they discovered a previously unknown signaling system that helps to regulate many body systems and functions. CB1 receptors are most concentrated in the brain and the central nervous system, though they are also found in other tissues and on cells in the immune system. CB2 receptors are found primarily in the peripheral organs and are known to influence immune function. This system of receptors throughout the body, along with the enzymes that synthesize and degrade endocannabinoids, was dubbed by researchers the ECS or endocannabinoid system. It appears that the function of the ECS is to help sustain homeostasis within our bodies. In other words the ECS helps to maintain harmony and balance between various body systems. Yoga, too, is designed to establish harmony in body, mind, and spirit, with equanimity and joy. The two share a compatibility of purpose and of effect.

At present we know that the ECS interacts with the nervous system, the immune system, the cardiovascular system, the respiratory system, the endocrine system, the reproductive system, and the digestive system. The ECS also has a direct influence on fertility, pain sensation, mood, appetite, memory, and bone growth. The cannabinoids are fundamentally anti-inflammatory. Because inflammation is part and parcel of every known degenerative disorder from diabetes to cancer to arthritis, this is of great value in reducing the risk of many types of disease.

From the earliest moments of development, to the last stages of life, your ECS is involved in constant mass communication with every organ system in your body, acting as the conductor in a symphony.

CARL GERMANO, *THE ROAD TO ANANDA*

The endogenous cannabinoids anandamide and 2-arachidonoyl-glycerol are produced as a result of the intake of dietary fats and oils. Specifically they result from a chemical cascade within the body that starts with omega-3 fatty acids, which are found in nuts and seeds and their oils, as well as in eggs, fish, and meat. But not everybody manufactures an adequate supply of inner cannabinoids, due to inefficient metabolism, poor quality dietary oils, and perhaps other metabolic causes as well. Cannabis expert and researcher Dr. Ethan Russo posits the hypothesis that many people may be fundamentally deficient in endocannabinoids. His paper "Clinical Cannabinoid Deficiency" delved into the various ways that cannabinoids function in the body and how a deficiency in cannabinoids can lead to a broad range of diseases. Taking off on this point, in 2010 I wrote an article for Fox News Health titled "Are You Cannabis Deficient?" The article was lavishly well received, and hundreds of readers thanked me for the information. An obvious answer to endocannabinoid deficiency is to supplement the body with exogenous cannabinoids (from outside sources), and there is no better source of cannabinoids on Earth than cannabis.

The phytocannabinoids (plant-derived cannabinoids) in cannabis directly activate the CB1 and CB2 receptors, thereby making up for a possible endocannabinoid deficiency. In this manner the cannabinoids, notably THC and CBD, act as vitamins. The true definition of a vitamin is something that our bodies require, other than minerals, which is either not made in the body or made in insufficient quantities yet is essential to health and life. Since the initial idea of cannabinoid deficiency was floated to the scientific community in 2001, researchers have established links between certain health disorders and low ECS function. In particular migraine headaches, PTSD, fibromyalgia, and irritable bowel syndrome are accompanied by low ECS function. When people with these disorders receive infusions of cannabinoids from cannabis, they enjoy more restful and satisfying sleep, experience decreased pain, and enjoy better overall quality of life. We need cannabinoids and our bodies generally respond very well to their consumption.

THC can bind to both CB1 and CB2 receptors, enabling it to exert influences throughout the body and mind. Because endocannabinoid receptors are the most concentrated neurotransmitter receptors in the brain, THC can and does deliver powerful mind-expanding effects. It is exactly because these effects are expansive that THC in cannabis enhances dimensions of yoga practice and sensation. CBD appears to behave differently from THC, not actually binding to receptors but keeping them active by other means, exerting influences on both CB1 and CB2 receptors. It is known to activate the 5HT1A (a serotonin receptor) and GPR55 receptor, which are also activated by anandamide. Non-psychotropic CBD is highly sought after for pain relief, for quelling nausea, and for improving sleep. In various cannabis-infused yoga classes around the United States, CBD infusion without THC is also very popular. Here I choose to focus on full-spectrum cannabis, containing both THC and CBD, for infusion as this is the practice that originated in the yoga tradition of India. If we are truly going to explore beyond our usual cognitive borders in our practice, then it is full-spectrum cannabis that acts as fuel in that endeavor.

As I have stated previously, the practice of yoga is largely a practice of the nervous system. With spinal flexibility and nerve elasticity at its heart, the active practices of yoga play endlessly upon the central nervous system. Cannabis, on the other hand, operates in the body through the ECS, the endocannabinoid system. These two, the nervous system and the ECS, meet and intertwine brilliantly when yoga is infused by cannabis. Cannabinoids signal to critically valuable neuroreceptors in the central nervous system including those for serotonin, acetylcholine, ATP, dopamine, GABA, and noradrenaline.

With the greatest number of neurosynaptic receptors in the brain, the ECS directly impacts executive function throughout the entire nervous system. Activity of the ECS in the brain, when properly supplied with a rich source of phytocannabinoids including THC and CBD, positively influences metabolism, growth and development, learning and memory, and other functions through a complex array of activities throughout the entire nervous system, from brain to toes. Yoga practice, as we know, enables the yogi to balance the systems of the body, quiet the mind, develop sharp powers of concentration, and gain control over various involuntary functions. Through yoga and meditation, one can significantly alter brainwave activity, entering into deep states of consciousness with increasing ease over time. The fusion of nerve enhancement and ECS activity in the central nervous system is the lotus and the bud, a seamless blend.

According to neuroscientists, our brains contain about one hundred billion neurons. The number of possible connections between them is said to exceed the number of atoms in the universe. Our habits of all types, including emotional habits and responses that do not serve us, are accompanied by well-established neural patterns. But when we practice yoga and meditate, and when we also infuse with cannabis, those habitual neurological pathways are suspended, at least temporarily, and new neural pathways arise. This enables us to more easily make new choices in thought, feeling, and deed, and to establish healthy neural patterns. This is the genius of the lotus and the bud, a neurobiological fusion that coordinates the effects and benefits of yoga with those of cannabis, in a manner that not only enhances and amplifies practice, but can help to alleviate anxiety, depression, PTSD, and other mood disorders. Both yoga and cannabis act as psychic lubricants, swinging wide open the doors of perception, and as potent medicines with the power to penetrate to the very core of a person and rewire their brains for the better.

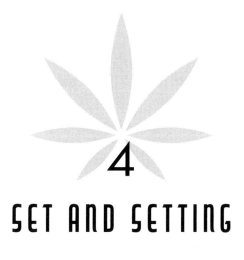

4

SET AND SETTING

GUIDELINES FOR PRACTICE

Establishing a time for daily practice is essential to embarking on a deep, cannabis-infused dive into yoga. After all there can be no practice if there is no time for it. There are three optimal times for practice. I personally think that the very best one is in the morning upon rising, because this allows you to jump-start your day with invigorating methods. Late in the afternoon seems to be another good time to practice. Most people are looser after a day of moving around. This can work to your advantage as you engage in flexibility-enhancing methods. Practicing at this time is also a refreshing punctuation to a day of work, especially if you need to go back and work for a few more hours. Setting aside time to practice in the evening caps off a busy day, and is often just what you need to clear your mind and ready yourself for deep, revitalizing sleep. This is a great way to work stress out of your body, and finish your day feeling centered, refreshed, and expanded.

Whatever your game plan make sure that you give yourself enough time to practice fully and completely, without rushing or cheating your routine. It may mean that you will surf the web less, or that you will need to cut back on some other activity. Modifying your schedule is just a natural part of making the changes necessary to go deeply into practice. Once you are in a regular flow of practicing, you will find that your new sense of energy, health, and well-being are well worth the changes you have made.

Specific Points of Advice on Practice

Take a shower or bath before practicing. This will loosen your body up considerably.

Practice when you have time. Do not hurry.

Practice on an empty stomach, not after a meal.

Practice in a place that is warm enough. Practicing in the cold can cause you to strain muscles.

Practice in a well-ventilated area. After all, breathing is very important!

Wear loose, nonrestrictive clothing. This will enable you to move freely.

When Not to Practice

If you are sick or badly injured, wait until you are better before resuming practice. If you are recovering from a debilitating chronic illness, take it easy. Practice is valuable and strengthening, but there are times when you must forgo it and rest. Respect the limits of your body. After all, we all have limits, and sometimes resting is the most beneficial thing you can do.

Don't Get Blasted

When you are ready to practice, by whatever means you are enjoying cannabis, do so in moderation. The idea is not to get blown to cosmic bits, but to expand awareness and enhance sensitivity to energy flow. Cannabis can enhance your capacity in yoga practice to move with fluidity through various states of mind and dimensions of consciousness with greater ease. It doesn't take much good cannabis to shift your internal condition. If you are vaporizing or smoking, a single hit or two will do the trick. If you are consuming cannabis chai or an edible, be moderate. In this manner cannabis acts as a psychic lubricant, an ease to practice. By contrast consuming a lot of cannabis prior to yoga can make practice difficult. The difference between intelligent application of cannabis and foolish application is the dose, and your attitude. Stoned yoga is just stoned yoga. Taking several bong hits or dabs prior to practice may in fact make yoga much harder to get through.

Finding your dose is fundamental to working with any and all psychoactive plants and fungi. Knowing what opens inter-dimensional doors in the psyche without getting too far out there is something everyone must figure out. As many manuals for products advise, your results may vary. We are each biologically and psychically unique. Our capacity and sensitivity to cannabis is individual. As you embark on yoga practice with cannabis, err on the gentle side. Remember that you can always have more. But once you have consumed too much, you can't have less.

INTENTION AND ATTENTION

What do you intend with your practice? What is your purpose? How do you bring yourself to the mat, to the moment, to the time that you set aside to engage in yoga, to open energy channels, and to dissolve the blockages that prevent full awareness of the spiritual self? I recommend that you bring yourself to practice with totality, humility, gratitude, reverence, and the earnest intention to surrender yourself to the great spirit of which we are part, from which we all derive, and which is all and everything. Practice is precious. Yoga is a gift to our lives, enhancing our conscious awareness, advancing our health, and tending us toward greater joy and happiness. Treat yoga practice as a special occasion.

Perhaps you intend to boost your health. Perhaps you intend to overcome notions and ideas that run counter to your happiness and integration. Perhaps you long to dissolve boundaries that blind you to the true interconnected nature of life, the fundamental oneness of everything. As you bring yourself to practice, reflect on your purpose. Clear mental space for engaging with yoga infused by cannabis. This is a set-aside time, not a time to sandwich between calls and emails. Your intentions may vary from day to day, depending on what is happening with you, your mood, your health, your emotional state. But, in any case, be intentional. Set a direction for yourself. This intention becomes a navigational polestar for practice.

Yoga helps us to develop greater attention to the moment, to the now, to the only thing that is actually taking place. Whatever is past is gone. Whatever future might exist has not come. Only the present is sure, and this is where we live. Most of the time the human condition is such that we mull over what has passed and turn our attention urgently to what may come. This leaves living right now out of the equation. And yet now is the only time that we live.

Be here now.
RAM DASS

I am not suggesting that reflecting on life or planning for the future lacks value or is unnecessary. But I am suggesting that yoga practice requires full presence. Bring yourself completely to the moment. Everything else that is happening in your life will still be happening. For practice pay attention to your breathing, your body sensations, the current of your thoughts as they flow along, the energy currents opening within you. Wherever you are, on a mat, a floor, a carpet, be there entirely.

The quality of your attention sets the course for your practice. If your thoughts drift, gently steer your attention back to the only thing that is happening, which is now. As you engage in practice, feelings and sensations and energy flow shift and change. Your task is to consciously ride the currents in which you find yourself, and which flow inside of you, and to stay tuned in. Managing your attention is a key to mastery. Concentrate on your yoga. Be fully present. Give yourself entirely to this.

FEELING AND VISUALIZING

I will share a secret that can significantly enhance your experience with yoga and cannabis. Many people advocate visualizing one thing or another, visualizing the chakras, visualizing energy flow, visualizing the third eye, and so forth. Without question, visualization is a valuable yogic tool. Tibetan Buddhist yogis, for example, learn to visualize brilliantly colorful geometric patterns, or yantras, down to the last detail. This practice helps them to develop superior mental concentration. But I will propose to you that concentrating on *feeling* provides a more rapid, easy means to awaken and amplify the flow of kundalini throughout our entire body-mind being. For while you may visualize the flow of kundalini up through the central channel of the spine, you can actually just plain feel that flow to some extent at any time.

Energy currents flow through us 24/7. They never stop. Energy hums through us, in neural activity, in fuel production in the mitochondria of our cells, in enzyme reactions, as brainwaves, cardiovascular rhythms, photon emissions, and electrical emissions in the nerve plexuses that align with the chakras, and through the spinal cord itself, the central channel. Instead of visualizing any of this energy, learn to feel it. As you pay attention in yoga, allow yourself to tune in to the myriad of sensations within you, and to follow the flow of energy in those sensations. We embody millions of energetic currents. You can put your attention at any one of the chakras, from muladhara at the base of the spine to sahasrara at the top of the head. Let go of all tensions and just feel that area, without any visualization. Pay attention to how that area feels. In fairly short order you will tap into the energy flow.

Getting into a deep flow of illuminating energy through feeling is one of the great yogic secrets. We are alive due to the currents of energy that run within us. And when those currents cease, we will be alive no more. Energy flow is everything. And we can feel energy.

This is where cannabis provides a very superb assist. As an amplifier and an activator, cannabis enables us to more readily experience subtle energies. This is a real technique, something to give special attention. If you put your attention at your spine, without visualizing anything at all, you will feel at least some subtle currents of sensation. By concentrating on those currents, they naturally amplify. And with cannabis they amplify more quickly and easily. This is due in part to the intertwining of two key internal biosystems, the nervous system and the endocannabinoid system.

I have found over my long years of yoga practice that feeling energy is a sure path to activating and amplifying kundalini flow. Learn to feel energy within and around you. Develop fine voluntary controls through diligent and uncompromising yoga practice and employ cannabis for activation and amplification.

MENTAL ATTITUDE

Here is an astonishing fact: The human brain contains approximately one hundred billion nerve cells, or neurons. Brain researchers have calculated that the possible number of interconnections that can be made between these neurons exceeds the number of total atoms in the universe! Ponder that for a moment. There is no easy way to imagine the fullness and complexity of the brain inside your head. The brain is vast, powerful, flexible, and virtually inexhaustible in terms of what it can do.

This vast, virtually inexhaustible brain is where the mind resides. Some people will take umbrage at the notion that the mind is anything other than a remarkable function of the brain, while others assert that mind is an emanation of a greater, unified conscious field, and that the brain is an ingenious device through which the mind acts. I fall squarely in the latter camp. While it would be a lively and entertaining exercise to go fifteen rounds pitting the neuro-reductionists of the former camp against the latter unified field group, it isn't necessary or purposeful to do so here, because the case I am making in this chapter doesn't require that you accept one version or another. But you might muse over what you think, and why. Are we all just remarkable neurology, or is each human being a conscious spirit inhabiting a physical body? This is a question that has resulted in more than a few red-faced shouting matches between academicians and philosophers. Are you simply an ingenious aggregation of blood, hair, and bones? Or are you spirit in flesh? It's a big question.

Just as your brain is incalculably diverse, so is your mind. Your mind is your vehicle to infinite possibilities. With your mind you can think, plan, dream, envision, and approach ideas and topics in myriads of ways. The human mind is spectacular, awesome, and greater than we can fully appreciate. And despite the attempts of psychologists, neurologists, chemists, and brilliant researchers of diverse fields to plumb the depths of human consciousness, we know only a fraction of what can be known. Our inquiries into the vastness of the mind are like the first halting, staggering steps of an awkward, diaper-clad toddler. We have a long, long way to go before we can claim that we have grasped the full nature and scope of the mind. Consider the works of the great artists, writers, poets, philosophers, inventors, explorers, adventurers, and leaders throughout history, and you can get an inkling of the mind's possibilities. The point is, the capacity for greatness and genius is built into us. If you are truly serious about embarking upon a program that will transform your health and revitalize your life, you need to bring the full focus and power of your mind to the task. Unless you are already actively engaged in a rejuvenation program, you are going to need to change your habits, restructure your time, and cultivate an attitude of success.

Therefore I'm going to introduce you to some fundamental mental steps that make it easy to cultivate the right attitude, achieve what you want, and become the master of your own destiny. Your path to superior health and balance will be easier to follow. In fact, any other endeavor will be easier, if you apply the same principles and practices. Remember this: Your mind is your friend. It is designed to serve you. You can sculpt and mold and shape the tendencies and habits of your mind to help you to fulfill your ambitions and realize your dreams. Your mind is the source of your personal power, and that power is immense.

Focusing Your Intent

A winning attitude starts with focused intent, a clear idea of what you want. While it is possible to achieve good things by random happenstance and plain dumb luck, it is a poor life strategy. You stand a much better chance of getting what you want if you know what you want and you chart a course for getting it. Do you want to be fit and healthy? If so, begin the process of getting what you want by defining exactly what fit and healthy means to you. Don't say to yourself, "I intend to get healthy and fit." That is vague and undefined. Instead, craft a specific language and vision of your goals. Focus your intent.

Let's say that you're inflexible in head-to-knee pose, and you're too stiff to bend forward all the way. Determine that through a daily practice you are going to go deeply into the pose, fully forward. Or let's say plank pose will help you with core strength. Set a goal to easily hold the pose for a minute or more, and practice until you are there. Then increase the time. These are realistic, attainable goals. Don't be afraid to set goals that cause you to do some real work. Nobody ever achieved greatness by setting timid goals. On the other hand don't go bananas setting goals that are wholly unattainable, either. When I introduce new students to yoga, I encourage the person who is determined to practice twenty minutes of yoga five days per week, and caution the person who announces that they are going to launch into a strenuous, three-hour daily practice for life. My experience is that usually the former student stands a much better chance of becoming involved with yoga for the long term. The latter individual wakes up one morning, realizes he's just committed himself to the equivalent of climbing Mt. Everest barefoot in skivvies, and gives up altogether. Push yourself, but don't go overboard. Any change worth making is worth making steadily and thoughtfully.

Having made a case for being sensible and moderate, it would be disingenuous of me to suggest that there is no room for fanatics. I started out practicing yoga for a couple of hours per day, and very quickly was engaged in eight hours or so of yoga and meditation daily. Fanatical? You bet. Recommended for most people? Not at all. But there is plenty of variety in the world. Some people really like to go charging into new things like bellowing war elephants. If that's your way, disregard my cautions and take it to the limit.

Once you have established your personal goals, continue to focus your intent. When are you going to practice? Whatever time you choose make that time sacred, and stick to it. My time is in the morning. Whether I'm at home, in a hotel, in the South Seas, or in the Himalayas, I practice then. Be willing to do whatever it takes to stay focused on your goals. In my decades of yoga and meditation, I have only been in one circumstance in which I could not engage in practice. I was in the Amazon during the flooded season, staying in a shack with a family of natives where there literally was no room to practice. I'm not telling you this to impress you, but to impress *upon* you the notion that focusing your intent means that you do not waver. Unless you encounter a circumstance (such as serious illness or injury) that absolutely prohibits you from doing what you have set out to accomplish, find a way.

The last part of focusing your intent is to describe to yourself, in clear, accurate language, exactly what you are going to accomplish, by what means and over the course of what period, and visualize yourself engaging in that process. See yourself practicing. See yourself achieving your goals.

Galvanizing Your Will

Once you have clearly identified your goals and aspirations, the next step is to galvanize your will. This is your sense of determination. If one-legged individuals can learn to ski double black diamond trails, can you accomplish less outlandish important goals with yoga? If common, everyday individuals can commit acts of great heroism, can you commit simple acts of integration and health? If millions of people every day can face life-threatening adversity and hardship, can you face the challenges of deep yoga practice? Think about it. Think hard. What does it take?

It takes a will forged in the flames of the desire to succeed. There is a saying that a warrior does not bow to a gale, he rides upon its crest. Becoming ever more accomplished in yoga practice is hardly like riding the crest of a howling gale, but at times it may well seem like it to you. Be determined to succeed. Be determined to do whatever it takes to be aware and open to the energies within and without, to be fit and healthy, to live your life in keen condition. Become galvanized. Feel yourself becoming immovably resolved, no compromise, no turning back, no waffling, no backing down. Talk yourself out of every reason you come up with to procrastinate, quit, or go soft. Just practice.

Being Congruent

You've set your goals, visualized your success, and forged a powerful sense of determined direction. So far so good. Now comes the follow-through, the time to be congruent, to think, feel, and act in a manner consistent with your intent. Being congruent is walking your talk. It's living up to your dreams and practicing what you espouse. This is what makes people vital and strong. With yoga, practice is it. There is practice and nothing else. All improvements, realizations, achievements, revelations happen through practice. Maybe you didn't expect some of this in a volume about yoga and cannabis. No matter what the specifics of your practice may be, in a hot room, on an airy porch, in a studio, on a boat dock, that is your time to harness your intention and your will, to give your practice strength and focus.

Positive Attitude

The pervasive ingredient through all of this mental cultivation is to remain positive in your attitude and approach to circumstances. Eventually a positive outlook on life becomes a consistent life-reinforcing habit. That in turn generates its own attractions, to positive people and outcomes. One of the benefits of yoga practice is inspiration. If you tap into the deep flow of energy in yoga, you will be inspired, uplifted. Yoga not only offers spectacular benefits to body, mind, and spirit, but it is a tremendous privilege. It is a bearer of illumination and joy.

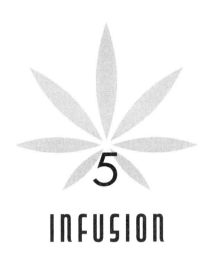

5

INFUSION

HOW TO INFUSE

Cannabis is a versatile plant, offering many ways to infuse your yoga. When I first started to become familiar with cannabis, there were two forms to enjoy, bud and hashish. Times were simpler. Now there is a large and ever-growing menu of widely available options. You have choices, varying from smoking bud or hash, to vaporizing either, to utilizing any of the various concentrates available. With bud or hashish, your choices are to smoke, to vaporize, or to consume in edibles. I describe both hashish and edibles in more thorough detail later.

The most common method of consuming bud remains the joint, a cigarette paper with cannabis rolled in it. Rolling papers can be made of standard wood pulp paper fiber, rice paper, hemp, bamboo, or other materials. When I began with cannabis in 1967 one of the most popular papers was made by Zig Zag from golden wheat straw. Smoking is not the healthiest way to infuse with cannabis, as you take in tars and other unwanted compounds in the smoke. But it is also the case that up to this point we know of no cases of cancer of the mouth, throat, larynx, bronchi, or lungs associated with cannabis. I confess that joints are still my favorite way to infuse, a holdover from my teens. You can crumble tiny bits of hash into a cannabis joint, and this of course amplifies the effects quite a lot. Caveat emptor.

Extracts

Extracts make up the remaining forms of cannabis available today. They are also widely called concentrates. Since you hear a lot about extracts in the cannabis scene, I'll give you the basics of what that means. Extraction as it applies to plants involves separating soluble materials (those that can be dissolved) from the insoluble cellulose plant skeleton. Plants are made largely of cellulose, which grows into an endless number of shapes and sizes. Woods, grasses, and fiber plants are all utilized for their cellulose. Inside the cells and walls of the cellulose, compounds of all kinds make up the chemistry of plants. Proteins, lipids, sugars, antioxidants, alkaloids, fats, waxes, and endless classes of compounds can be found in plants. The idea of extraction is to remove the soluble compounds from the cell walls of the plant as efficiently as possible, leaving behind only inert cellulose material. The temperature of extraction, the solvents used, and many other methods determine this efficiency.

When you make a cup of tea, you perform basic hot water extraction. Dried tea leaves are cut into small particles, breaking open the plant cell walls. When freshly boiled water is poured onto the tea, the soluble materials in the plant cell walls leak out, transforming the color of the water, and conveying flavor and aroma thanks to hundreds of naturally occurring compounds. When you make a cup of drip coffee from freshly ground beans, the process and method are basically the same as with tea, employing hot water to extract the flavor and biologically active compounds like caffeine and its chemical cousins. Espresso forces steam at pressure through very finely ground coffee, resulting in a heavy, rich, concentrated coffee extract. On an industrial scale, herbs, spices, flavoring agents, and cooking oils of all kinds are extracted in massive quantities, typically with many tons of material in a single batch. The extracts and oils will go into foods, beverages, and household products from cleaners to air fresheners to tobacco. We consume extracts all the time.

All that said extraction with cannabis is actually quite different from extraction of other plants. This is because the cannabinoids and terpenes from cannabis reside outside of the plant cell walls, as little glands of resin. To make virtually all cannabis extracts, except for the alcohol extract described later, it is not necessary to break open the cell walls of the plant. Due to this unique composition of cannabis, the idea of extraction is to separate the resin from the rest of the plant by dissolving it from the surface of the buds and sugar leaves. Resin is soluble in alcohol, and thus alcohol makes a good extraction solvent for cannabis. Resin is also soluble in fats and oils, which I describe in the section on edibles.

Not all cannabis concentrates are clean. Many are made with either butane or propane, the same gasses used in cigarette lighters and home heating. While highly efficient as solvents, these gasses are also toxic. There is simply no reason to use products extracted with toxic solvents when cleaner versions are so readily available. Among the many concentrates on the market, the preferred ones made without toxic solvents are CO_2 oil, bubble hash, rosin, and Phoenix Tears.

CO_2 Oil

Made by extracting the resin of cannabis under pressure with pure carbon dioxide, CO_2 oil is super concentrated and clean. In dispensaries you will often find amber-colored CO_2 extract sold in syringes, not for injection but for controlled application in recipes.

Bubble Hash

A simple hashish made by separating plant material from resin using ice water, bubble hash is as clean as it gets. You can make bubble hash at home if you have enough plant material. Plus, by making your own you will know what strain is used, which often is not the case when you acquire concentrates.

Rosin

Clean and golden, rosin is made by pressing cannabis buds between hot plates, melting the resin from the trichomes and draining it from the plant matter. This method can be performed for a very small amount using a hair straightener.

Phoenix Tears

An invention of Rick Simpson, who is famous for helping many people with health problems with Rick Simpson Oil. Distilled with pure alcohol and dark in color, Phoenix Tears is also typically sold in a syringe for controlled application.

Vapor Cartridges

Vapor cartridges typically contain propylene glycol, a slightly sweet syrup that was never ever meant to be heated and inhaled into the lungs. Vapor cartridges for both tobacco and cannabis are demonstrating serious health risks, and already we have seen some bans of vapor cartridges. Yes, cartridges and vapor pens are super convenient. But using them can coat your lungs with goo and obstruct your respiration. Stay away from them.

Alcohol Extracts (tinctures)

Liquid extracts, or tinctures, of cannabis are made using pure alcohol as a solvent. Liquid extracts involve cooking whole buds in pure grain alcohol, and that does in fact result in pulling the soluble materials out of the cannabis cell walls in addition to separating the resin from the buds. This results in a green, astringent, and tasty fluid that can be put into an oral spray bottle, or dropper-top bottle. Clean and rapid in effect, alcohol extracts are convenient to carry and use.

Unfortunately the federal government applies such an extraordinary tax to pure alcohol that it is virtually unaffordable in comparison with toxic butane and propane.

Butane and Propane Concentrates

Concentrates made with either butane or propane are simply not healthy products. And while advocates of such an extraction method will claim that all residues of butane or propane are evaporated from the final concentrate, residues always remain. Why pollute your body with industrial fuels? The following widely available concentrates are off my recommended list exactly because they are made with these solvents.

Shatter: Typically extracted with the solvent butane, shatter appears like porous semitransparent amber glass, and easily breaks into fragments. Beautiful to look at, popular, and versatile, shatter is a nonstarter because of its toxic means of manufacture.

Live Resin: Not to be confused with rosin, live resin is made with butane extraction of frozen plant material. Forget it.

Crumble, Wax, and Butter: Crumble, wax, and butter are also made with butane or propane. Forget them.

Tools of Reverie

Vaporizers

Vaporizers, not to be confused with vapor cartridges, are vastly popular, and for good reasons. With many vaporizers you can use bud, hash, bubble hash, rosin, Phoenix Tears, or CO_2 oil. A vaporizer heats up the cannabis until the resin turns into a vapor or gas. This vapor is inhaled, not smoke. Vaporizing is quick and easy and produces a rapid effect. Vaporizers vary in terms of technicality of use. Some are very simple to operate, while others offer a more complex menu of functions than you may want.

Pipes, Bongs, Nargilehs

The equipment available for smoking cannabis and its preparations ranges from simple corncob pipes to blowtorch-heated "dabbing pipes" made of thick, tempered glass.* The basic idea of any pipe or piece of smoking gear is to enable the user to quickly and readily infuse with smoke. My personal preferences tend to run to low-tech simple pipes, no blowtorches. One of the simplest pipes of all is the chillum, a conical pipe typically made of clay. Popular in India and Nepal, chillums are held upright in the hand, so you actually smoke through a chamber made with your palms.

One of the most iconic pieces of cannabis smoking equipment is

---

*Dabbing is a form of vaporizing that basically uses a high-tech glass pipe and a blowtorch (yes for real) to vaporize a resinous concentrate and take in a huge amount of psychoactive material in one breath. In my estimation this is total overkill, too much too fast.

the bong. A glass filtration device, a bong allows you to smoke cannabis filtered through water, producing a cooler and cleaner smoke. Bongs vary in size and cost, from small simple affairs to large and ornate hand-blown glass works of art.

From antiquity we have the nargileh or hookah, a water tobacco pipe that originated in the Near East also very commonly used for hashish. As with a bong, a nargileh uses water filtration. You smoke with a mouthpiece through a hose attached to the reservoir of the device, drawing in smoke á la *The Arabian Nights* or the caterpillar in *Alice in Wonderland*. Many nargilehs are ornately decorated, with colorful striped hoses and sometimes ornate glass work, and may have one or more hoses attached. In the Middle East the nargileh, or *qalyan* as it is also known, has a long history of use for smoking hashish. As that region is a hashish breadbasket and availability has historically been of little concern, it is not unreasonable for one or two people to pick up the hoses of a nargileh and happily work their way through smoldering coal-sized chunks of fragrant regional hash.

If you choose to infuse by any of the means described above, keep in mind all rules of safety and personal tolerance. Infusing with cannabis for yoga is itself an act of practice. Be thoughtful, caring, and attentive to the moment. Figure out what works best for you, what gives you the right assist with yoga and with diving deeply into the cosmic current to which we are all connected.

CANNABIS CONFECTIONS, ELECTUARIES, AND BAKED GOODS

If you think back to the tale about Siva eating cannabis, you have an important piece of information about this plant. For while cannabis acts most quickly upon the body and mind when smoked or vaporized, it acts most profoundly when it is eaten. For this reason many writers and poets have waxed effusive at the astonishing ecstasies of eating cannabis, especially in its most concentrated form as hashish. In potency of effect smoked cannabis pales in comparison to cannabis eaten. Taking the cannabinoids into your body via the respiratory system is quick and popular. But absorbing cannabinoids into the digestive tract takes a bit more time and produces a longer and potentially stronger effect. With edibles you can either enjoy a mild and leisurely lift in mood, or you can strap yourself into your seat and go full psychedelic. For our purposes we'll stay on the mild and leisurely lift side.

Edibles have been with us for a long, long time. Back in the 1980s I acquired an original sixteen-volume edition of Sir Richard Francis Burton's translation of *Alf layla wa layla*, or *One Thousand and One Nights*, known most commonly as *The Arabian Nights*. Tales from *The Arabian Nights* trace back to the eighth century, and stories in that collection derive from Arabic, Persian, Jewish, Turkish, Greek, and Indian folklore. The collection of tales derives not from one author but from many storytellers, merchants, travelers, writers, scholars, and others stretching back at least many centuries prior to the first publication. In one of the sixteen volumes I found a footnote about *ma'jun*, a type of cannabis electuary or confection, also known as majoun or majoon. It turns out that majoun recipes vary and may include cannabis-infused butter or oil, honey, and dried fruits, nuts, and spices, all chopped finely and worked together and made into either fingers or balls. Exceptionally tasty, majoun is one of those confections that captivates with both its rich and sumptuous flavor and its magic-carpet effects. Celestial and enlivening, majoun opens the realms of the human imagination easily and seemingly magically. It is a time-consuming recipe to make well, but an extraordinary treat when made with great care. For infused yoga a small ball or finger of majoun is pretty much without compare for putting you in an amplified and extra-inspired zone.

In India . . . Ma'jun (= electuary, generally) is made of ganja or young leaves, buds, capsules, and florets of hemp (C. sativa), poppy-seed, and flowers of the thorn-apple (datura) with milk and sugar-candy, nutmegs, cloves, mace, and saffron, all boiled to the consistency of treacle which hardens when cold.
FOOTNOTE IN THE TALE OF ALA AL-DIN ABU AL-SHAMAT,
THE ARABIAN NIGHTS

I would discourage anybody from making the recipe as described by Burton with the inclusion of datura, as that plant contains the tropane alkaloids atropine, scopolamine, and hyoscyamine, which can disorient or even kill you. The tropane alkaloids are powerful and unfriendly hallucinogens, producing spooky or outright terrifying visions. In fact both datura and its botanical cousin brugmansia have long been employed for robbery and murder. Majoun surely needs no datura to provide extraordinary effects.

In *The Cannabis Kitchen Cookbook* by Robyn Griggs Lawrence, I contribute a majoun recipe, so I will not reproduce one here. But suffice it to say that the majoun deriving from that recipe is almost too delicious, and I encourage you to make and try it. Robyn's book is sensational. It's pretty much the standard-bearer for cannabis cookery, and if you are going to infuse with your own edibles then it's the go-to volume. In that book you'll also find my inspiring Good Morning Sativa Chai, which is a remarkably easy way to infuse and has a very rapid effect.

Among these sweets is a kind of electuary made with the fatty extract (of hashish), figs, dates and honey. Another very popular kind, madjoun, has cloves, cinnamon, pepper, musk, and other similar substances. It is said to be highly stimulating.

BARON ERNST VON BIBRA

The cannabinoids in cannabis are most soluble in a fat of some kind. For this reason butters and oils are essentials of cannabis cookery. Make a cannabis butter and that material can be employed in a vast variety of baked goods and confections. So, too, infused oils lend themselves to quick and easy use. Oils help our bodies to absorb the cannabinoids through the gut. Whether you follow a traditional Ayurvedic approach and infuse ghee with cannabis or you are vegan and infuse coconut oil, the idea is to get the cannabis into a form that will be best utilized by the body. Cannabis plus oil equals excellent absorption and maximum effect.

While virtually any recipe, from nachos to tiramisu, can be made with cannabis, edibles suitable for infusing yoga practice occupy a somewhat narrower band. A morsel of cookie, brownie, or chocolate or a cup of chai or infused coffee can all serve well as ample sacraments for your journey through yoga. By comparison cannabis lasagna is less suitable, as it is too much food for practice. Keep it light, easy, and simple. I'm a big fan of chai or infused coffee. Both work well and quickly. Whatever you choose, savor that. Put your attention into it and appreciate your communion with the spirit of cannabis.

Electuaries are sweet and often flavored with spices. Electuaries are the preferred medicinal doses in the Middle Eastern traditional medicine systems like *Unani*, where honey and sugar preparations have long been the vehicles for medicinal formulas of all kinds. They may be formed into pills, balls, fingers, or pastilles of various sorts. An electuary of cannabis would typically blend a cannabis butter or oil with some honey or sugar. This type of preparation was consumed in the famous Club des Haschichins in Paris and contained fat, honey, and pistachios. The paste was known as *dawamesk*. Like majoun, dawamesk is a type of regional electuary for which recipes vary. Deriving from North Africa, dawamesk appears as a greenish spread similar to jam and may contain hashish, butter, honey, sugar, pistachio, cinnamon, clove, or nutmeg. The writers who consumed dawamesk at Club des Haschichins were likely eating an electuary of Algerian hash. Algeria was a hot spot for adventurous travelers on the hunt for unique experiences and was a hashish breadbasket. The flow of travelers between the cities of Europe and Algeria ensured an equally good flow of hashish from that North African country.

Making your own confections is relatively easy and provides another opportunity to get close to cannabis, to work with it, to make something from it. And if you enjoy trying out new ideas in the kitchen as I do, then making confections, baked goods, and drinks is a lot of fun. When my wife, Zoe, and I went out to Colorado for a day of cooking and a photo shoot for *The Cannabis Kitchen Cookbook*, we all had a blast making and trying seven recipes. My day started on a solid foundation of yoga, coffee, and breakfast, and that helped me to keep the stamina required to survive testing all our foods and drinks. There is certainly nothing wrong with purchasing ready-made products. But know your sources and their ingredients. If you make your own confections or baked goods, you know everything about what went into them. That is a great advantage. Pure organic confections without unwanted additives go along best with the purifying, cleansing, healing, and restorative effects of yoga practice.

How much is wise to consume? Of course everybody is so different one from another that there are no clear guidelines, but it is best to err on the lower potency side. You can always have more, but you can never have less. If you are making your own edibles, learn to calibrate amounts of ganja to servings. With high-quality cannabis flower, about one-third of a gram is a good amount for a single drink, confection, or electuary. In the case of hashish, reduce that to one-sixth of a gram or even less. Remember that there are twenty-eight grams to an ounce. So one-fourth of an ounce would be seven grams. A brownie mix with that much cannabis bud would yield twenty-one or so brownies. Whatever you make, perform a bio-assay; that is, try it yourself, prior to offering it to others. If you are going to give someone else a cannabis confection you should know its potency and effects first. For me this is an inviolable principle.

Maximizing Cannabis Potency

In 1970 the U.S. government cannabis program head Dr. Norman Doorenbos of the University of Mississippi and his team made a potent discovery. When cannabis is heated to 100°C for ninety minutes, the carboxyl radical is broken off of tetrahydrocannabinolic acid (THCA), producing THC, tetrahydrocannabinol, and the pot becomes far more potent. Nifty trick. What this means is that you can transform moderately potent ganja into appreciably more potent material by heating it properly.

This process is known today as decarboxylation, or "decarbing." By heating cannabis at approximately 212 to 220°F for about forty-five minutes, you can convert THCA into THC. This is commonly performed in order to smoke or vaporize cannabis, making it stronger. But with those cannabis recipes that are cooked, no prior decarboxylation is necessary. When you cook cannabis butter or oil, or bake brownies, cakes, etc., the heat involved accomplishes the task of decarbing.

Ultimate Ganja Cookies

This recipe is for the very finest cannabis cookies in the world. These cookies are not only sensationally delicious and nutritious, but they infuse the mind and body with the reveries of Siva's benefic vibrations.

1 stick of butter

¼ to ½ ounce finely ground cannabis (I highly recommend powdering the cannabis in a coffee grinder)

½ cup pure maple syrup

1 cup almonds, ground in a blender into coarse flour

1/3 cup oatmeal, ground in a blender into coarse flour

1/3 cup shredded, dried coconut

1/3 cup wheat germ

1 cup pastry flour

¼ teaspoon powdered cinnamon

a pinch of salt

Place the stick of butter in a pan and melt at low heat. When the butter is thoroughly melted, stir in the finely ground cannabis and simmer it in the butter at low heat for 10 to 15 minutes. This oil simmering process is probably the single most important part of preparation. Next, remove the cannabis butter from the stove and add the maple syrup to it. Stir thoroughly. Combine all the other ingredients in a bowl. Then mix the butter-cannabis-syrup mixture into the dry ingredients with a spoon.

When the ingredients are thoroughly mixed, fashion between 24 and 36 dome-shaped cookies, and lay them out on a cookie sheet. Bake at 350°F for 10 to 12 minutes, until golden brown. Cool and serve.

Caution: These cookies taste extremely delicious. They are remarkably healthy, too. But remember, they are ganja cookies. It's always best to start with less, as you can consume more if you choose. Do not make the mistake of eating a whole bunch at once, as you will be truly hammered and begging for divine relief. Yoga is the last thing you would want to do. You should feel the effects within forty-five minutes. But wait at least an hour and a half before making the decision to consume more. Don't munch on them like chips. Eat one, or maybe just half of one.

>✣〜✣<

At some point during a leisurely idyll on the island of Jamaica, I hopped onto a red Honda motor scooter and weaved my way through bustling traffic into the center of town toward the legendary Miss Brown's in Negril. The morning had involved a swim, yoga, coffee, and breakfast of Jamaica's deservedly famous fresh tropical fruit. A few days prior I had tried Jenny's special chocolate cannabis cake up on the cliffs near where I was staying, and enjoyed a pleasant afternoon on the cliffs and in the undulating waters of the Caribbean. But Miss Brown's was by all accounts the place to go for the finest cannabis cake on the island. Pretty much everybody said so.

After successfully navigating Negril traffic without mishap, I found myself at Miss Brown's perusing a menu of psychoactive offerings, from mushroom tea to brownies. "You ever have Miss Brown's cake?" asked the young man with whom I spoke. I explained that no, I hadn't, but I had tried the cake at Jenny's. He looked me dead in the eye. "Nobody, I mean nobody, makes the cake like Miss Brown."

It sounded like the kind of line delivered before a shoot-out in a Western, as though Miss Brown had harnessed the mighty elemental forces of all nature. I ordered a piece of cake to go. The young man nodded, suggesting I had made a wise choice.

Back on the cliffs I thought to start moderately by eating only half the piece of cake with a glass of fresh fruit juice. Properly prepared, cannabis works remarkably quickly when eaten, and I had not waited for even half an hour when the first tremulous inklings of psychedelic liftoff tickled my nerves. I was seated in a comfortable chaise longue, and thrilling sensations pulled my spine upright; my eyes opened more widely and my awareness began to expand rapidly. It was a fast takeoff out onto the vast jet-streams of the mind. I could hear every bird along the rocky Negril cliffs, could smell dozens of scents mingling in a soft ocean breeze, and could see the most subtle shadings of colors in the trees, water, buildings, and environment around me. I was soaring.

I brought my attention to the base of my spine, where I felt pressure building. A stream of energy, bright and expansive, flowed smoothly up through me, streaming out the top of my head. In my mind's eye I saw a bright light surrounding me and expanding in all directions, mingling with every atom in the atmosphere. My cells felt bathed in light. Throughout my body I felt as though fine electrical currents were streaming through tissues, organs, bones. My nostrils felt like tunnels, and the breath blowing through them seemed like a wind from the farthest depths of antiquity. I rode that vast, expansive, mysterious current for the better part of an hour, absorbed in cosmic energy.

My senses went into overdrive. Later when I dove into the undulating pearlescent blue water of the sea, my body dissolved like sugar. When I sat in the sun, the heat baked my bones and crackled along every nerve. When I sipped some fine Jamaican Blue Mountain coffee, the smell and taste of all the lush, green vegetation and fruit trees and creeping vines and giant-leafed exotic plants and soft, loamy, rich soil filled my mouth and nose. I was on a journey to the far horizon of consciousness, and my part was to take delight in the ride.

>~~~~~<

A shock, as of some unimagined vital force, shoots without warning through my entire frame, leaping from my fingers' ends, piercing my brain, startling me till I nearly spring from my chair.

FITZHUGH LUDLOW, *THE HASHEESH EATER*

HASHISH, THE GREAT YOGIC SACRAMENT

Though you face many good choices of forms of cannabis for infusing for your yoga practice, my favorite of all is hashish. For purity, fragrance, and delightful effect, nothing else comes close. Perhaps my personal affinity for hashish comes from my days in boarding school, when I was introduced to Lebanese blond hash by a fellow student whose father was posted in a diplomatic capacity in Beirut. I can conjure the exact fragrance in my imagination to this day. Hashish can be considered the crème de la crème of cannabis, the peak of the cannabis aficionado's art. Today there are many well-described and clever ways of producing hashish, from dry sift to bubble hash. The web has endless numbers of demonstration videos for making your own hashish, should you possess the volume of raw material (cannabis buds) and the will to do so. However it is more likely that you will acquire hashish. And as there are many varieties from which to choose, the hashish experience resembles that of coffee, chocolate, or wine. Good hashish conveys the unique characteristics of the cannabis from which it is made, the variations of which are almost innumerable. In each case you can select from the fragrance, flavor, and effects that you appreciate the most. As a sacrament, hashish is ideal, offering concentrated mood-modifying benefits quickly, getting you readily into a fine flow ideally suited for yogic immersion. It has been my great good fortune to experience hashish in numerous temples in the Kumaon region of India, up in the Himalayan hills, where the sacrament is made and highly valued.

At the Someshwar Mahadev Mandir Temple outside of Almora in the Kumaon district of the Indian Himalayas, the priest Gopal Giri Mahatma invited me to join in the worship of Siva. "Smoking?" he asked, fingering a mala of bodhi seeds and leaning toward me on the worn tiger skin where he sat. I nodded yes, replying that I would be happy to join him. From a vest pocket he produced a folded piece of paper in which he kept pieces of charas, the local handmade hashish. Gopal Giri Mahatma handed the charas to me along with a bidi, a cigarette of tobacco wrapped in a tendu leaf. I emptied the bidi of tobacco and filled it carefully with tiny crumbled pieces of hash. The priest may have expected me to mix the hash with tobacco from the cigarette, but I chose instead to construct a cleaner sacramental smoke, somewhat more painstakingly, without.

"Om Siva," the priest offered as I lit the ganja. I replied in kind, invoking the god of yoga and cannabis and spirit. In a temple setting the enjoyment of cannabis is always somewhat ceremonial, though not necessarily solemn. It is a set-aside time for reverie, a pause to pay attention to spirit. Preparing the charas respectfully, invoking Siva, and sitting in peace as we enjoyed the expansion that ensued was all ceremony. Candles flickered on an altar, incense wafted in the air. We sat together and smoked, and then passed a pleasant hour or so by the altar in the shade of some deodar trees as birds fluttered about and a small dhuni, or holy fire, burned near us. At the entrance to

the temple grounds, a steel cable hung with bells was shaken by each visitor, announcing to the gods that they had arrived upon the scene.

>᠇᠊᠊᠊᠇<

This scene is repeated in Himalayan temples every day. Priests and pilgrims sit together, take holy communion in the form of charas, and bask in the grace of Siva. The difference between the sacrament of charas at that temple and the grape juice and bread squares served at communion where I attended church as a youth could not be more stark. In the case of the latter, we imagined something as part of a story from antiquity. In the case of the charas sacrament, we enjoy a direct exalted experience. This is the case with both cannabis and yoga. They are experiential. You know them by their direct effects.

In the Nepalese and Indian Himalayas, hashish is a popular form of cannabis associated with yoga and the god Siva. The Kumaon hill region in particular is a stronghold of charas making and use, and the smoking of charas as a sacrament to the god Siva goes many centuries back in time. Throughout other parts of India, yogis and sadhus smoke cannabis flower, generally referred to as bhang and commonly mixed with tobacco. But hashish occupies a noble place in the yogic tradition. Fragrant, concentrated, and potent in effect, hashish is made by collecting and pressing the resin glands of mature female cannabis flowers. Hashish is made by various methods that have been developed over time in different regions. I confess an affection for hashish above all other forms of cannabis and am delighted by its aromas.

In the Himalayan foothills of India and Nepal, collectors run their hands up and down against the resinous flowers of mature flowering female plants, until their palms are covered with resin. They then rub their hands vigorously together to clump the resin into little balls. These little balls are rubbed together into larger balls, or into "fingers" of a regional hashish called charas. This charas is fragrant and sweet, with a floral aroma, and conveys a pleasant, lively high. This method of making hashish is likely the first method ever devised. Charas is made with pride. This is a jewel of the Himalayas, and many makers work hard to produce a superior and delightful product. Consistency, creaminess, delightful flavor, arresting aroma, and inspiring effect are all indicators of very well made charas.

The landmark *Report of the Indian hemp Drugs Commission 1893–1894* described the making of charas this way: "The female plants, having been cut in November, are spread out to dry for twenty-four hours. The people then sit around in the heat of the day, and pluck off the flower heads, which are now full of seed, discarding the coarser leaves. Each handful is rubbed between the palms for about ten minutes and thrown aside. In the course of time a quantity of juice accumulates on the palms, which is scraped off and rolled into balls. These are charas. Sometimes the plants are trodden instead of handled and the feet scraped. A more uncommon method, by which a choice kind of charas is obtained, is to pass the hands up the ripe plants while they are still standing in the field."

As exotic as the hand-rubbing method of hashish production may seem, it is inefficient, and best suitable for those instances in which there is a generously large amount of available ganja. This is the case in the Indian and Nepalese Himalayan foothills, where the yards of homes commonly feature a plot of cannabis for making charas. The people in that region enjoy a super abundance of high-quality cannabis. From what I have seen, the Himalayan cannabis is tall, with very large floral colas. The fragrance of those fully mature buds is evocative and complex, at once a blend of fresh sweet flowers and husky resins. I have found myself simply smelling fresh buds there, as the aroma is captivating.

English botanist and mycologist Mordecai Cooke also described the making of charas, and his account became oft-repeated for its evocative visuals. The comedy group Firesign Theatre would subsequently parody Cooke's account in one of their albums of the 1960s. "In Central India, the hemp resin called *churrus,* is collected during the hot season in the following manner. Men clad in leathern dresses run through the hemp fields, brushing through the plants with all possible violence; the soft resin adheres to the leather, and is subsequently scraped off and kneaded into balls . . . "

By far the most common production of hashish is accomplished by sieving. In this method ripe cannabis plants are harvested and dried, usually by hanging them upside down. When the plants are well dried, they are then shaken or lightly beaten against a fine sieve, through which the tiny resin glands fall. This results in a pile of fine, dust-like resin, which is highly malleable and easily molded at room temperature. The resin may be rolled into balls by hand, hammered into concentrated blocks, or mechanically pressed into squares. Some hashish is even stamped with a seal of origin. I remember Afghani hashish at college in the 1970s stamped with a brilliant gold seal of the Afghan resistance. It seemed almost too pretty to smoke. But that was a passing notion.

A pipe of kif in the morning gives one more strength than 100 camels in the courtyard.

MOROCCAN PROVERB

One method of hashish manufacture involves beating mature, dried cannabis plants against coarse carpet before sieving or sieving through fine cloth so that the resin glands of the flowers are shaken off onto the carpet. Subsequently a piece of wooden board with sharp edges is scraped against the carpet surface to aggregate the resin. The important part of the process is that as much resin as possible is collected, and after that, any pieces of leaf or other debris, however fine, are removed by putting the resin through a fine sieve. High-quality hashish is free of debris and leaf material, contains no mold, is uniform in color and texture, and is malleable in the hand at room temperature.

Different types of hashish come from different regions. The legendary Nepalese Temple Ball and Manali cream varieties, both from Himalayan hill regions, are black and smooth. Hashish from the Beqaa Valley in Lebanon is typically reddish blond, and smells like no other hash in the world. Most Afghani hash is greenish brown. Some Middle Eastern hashish is blond or pink. Hashish from Northern California is typically pale green. Whatever the type or the origin, the goal of any real quality maker of hashish is to produce a uniform product made solely from resin glands, to ensure purity and potency. The resulting product must generate a delightful high and promote feelings of satisfaction and pleasure.

Hashish is most commonly either smoked in a pipe or eaten. As a smoke it is typically pleasant and lofty. As an eaten material it can be wildly powerful, a full-thundering psychedelic. For this reason you should approach the eating of hashish with care and caution. And if you are going to eat hash, cook it. Hashish can be made in conditions where hygiene and sanitation are poor or simply lacking. Innumerable pathogenic bacteria can and do reside in hash. You can become very sick from these bacteria. *E. coli* and other pathogenic microbes can produce fever, diarrhea, chills, vomiting, and even hallucinations if the bacterial load is heavy enough. If you wish to consume hashish orally in any form of preparation but have not made the hashish yourself, take care. Cook it to kill any germs.

Not being used to hashish . . . he burst into extraordinary hilarity and filled the hall with shouts of laughter.
THE TALE OF THE HASHISH EATER,
THE ARABIAN NIGHTS

In some places you can find hashish oil. This is a product made by extracting the oily cannabinoids from hashish with either alcohol or hydrocarbon solvents. I first encountered hash oil in Kathmandu in the early '80s. Depending on whether or not filtration is part of the procedure, the resulting oily goo can be black or even amber colored, as in the so-called honey oil of Nepal. Hash oil has caught on due in part to vaping technology and to dabbing, which involves using a blowtorch to heat a heavy tempered glass pipe to flaming red then swishing a bit of oil in the glowing hot bowl and sucking in the resulting vapor. This is extremely potent and not my style at all. I find good, well-made hashish consistently more fragrant and enjoyable, and far simpler to use. Plus, I do not want to support the use of toxic aromatic hydrocarbons like butane or benzene for any purpose, especially for making or enjoying a consumable item.

All things considered hashish is the cognac of ganja products. Throughout much of India, Nepal, Kashmir, Afghanistan, Turkey, and the Middle East, hashish is the preferred form of cannabis. This is owing to its rarefied nature and exquisite effects. A Sufi saying declares, "No wine or other tonic could generate such a heavenly sensation." In the three volume classic *The Great Books of Hashish* by Laurence Cherniak, the author says a most remarkable thing. "The hashishin (one who enjoys hashish) believes that with hashish you will be purified and placed in the center of all the world's immortal glory." This is the essential purpose of hashish as it relates to yoga practice. There is this sense of splendor, of magnificence and great beauty in hashish descriptions, of "heavenly sensation." It combines brilliantly well with the "heavenly sensation," generated by yoga and achieving mindfulness, a mixture of expansion, openness, joy, relief, oneness with the all and the everything. Enjoyed judiciously along the path to ever greater consciousness, hashish is an ally that can amplify the expansive fruits of practice.

I advise any bashful young man to take hashish when he wants to offer his heart to any fair lady, for it will give him the courage of a hero, the eloquence of a poet, the ardor of an Italian.

LOUISA MAY ALCOTT, *PERILOUS PLAY*

Taken moderately, hashish cheers a person's mind, and at most, perhaps, induces him to untimely laughing. If larger doses are taken, producing the so-called fantasia, we are seized by a delightful sensation that accompanies all the activities of our mind. It is as if the sun were shining on every thought passing through our brain, and every movement of our body is a source of delight.

JACQUES-JOSEPH MOREAU, M.D.

GROW YOUR OWN, KNOW YOUR OWN

If you are located in a state where the personal cultivation of cannabis is legal, then I advise you strongly to grow your own. My wife and I live in Massachusetts, where every household is allowed to grow a total of a dozen plants. Few people in our area grow that much cannabis for personal use, as the yield would be massive if the plants are well tended. Four or so plants per season can provide a large quantity of homegrown. Growing your own cannabis is relatively easy, and the rewards are great. First and foremost you get to start cannabis plants, and tend them to maturity. This is a delightful activity that does not require loads of work. As you go through this process, you learn about the plant. Cannabis is a hardy plant, and it is versatile as well. You can find excellent seeds online and can select the strains you want. I prefer to grow bright, lively sativa strains like Pine Warp and Kali Mist. In the parlance of the cannabis scene, even though all cannabis is *Cannabis sativa,* there is a lot of differentiation between expansive high sativa cultivars, and somewhat heavier indica cultivars. As I described earlier, there really is no such thing as indica. But those cannabis strains promoted as indica typically convey a more potent body effect, whereas those sold as sativa tend to be more bright and lively.

Today you can learn the basics of cannabis cultivation easily online. Many sites offer helpful advice on cultivation for the home grower. Armed with that knowledge, seeds, great soil and fertilizer materials, and the right sized pots or a good garden plot, you can grow your own and step out of much of the turbulent and increasingly corporate cannabis market. As a strong advocate of organic cultivation, I urge you to grow clean and green, never applying harmful agripoisons to your cannabis. There is absolutely nothing you can't do safely and naturally. Soil adjuncts like worm castings, bat guano, various mycorrhizae, lobster mulch, and other natural fertility builders can help you to grow strong, healthy, high-yielding plants right at home. And if you encounter pest issues, neem oil and other natural agents will send the bugs packing.

There is another aspect to growing your own as it relates to the blending of yoga and cannabis. As you work with your plants, put

yourself in a clear, open state. I will sometimes smoke a bit of cannabis before tending to my plants. In any case send your healthy, positive intentions to your plants. Talk to them. Groom them and make sure they lack for nothing. If you do this you will develop a rapport with the spirit of the plant, opening up an energetic portal that leads to further rich spiritual discovery. Initially this may seem like fantasy or imagination. But if you are diligent in your attention to your cannabis plants, you can experience a heightened state of awareness and an energetic interchange with your plants. All the good energy that you share with your plants translates into a close bond with your cannabis when harvest time comes.

When cannabis has reached full maturity and maximum bud growth, it is ready for harvesting. The main stalk is cut, as with chopping down a tree. The cannabis is usually dried by hanging the plants upside down. When the plants are dry, the lateral branches are cut from the main stalk, and the buds and leaf material are picked from those.

With commercial cannabis trimming is a key aspect of post-harvest processing. People do not want to consume stems and stalks. Nor should they. For this reason trimmers cut the buds and leaves of the cannabis away from branch and stem material. This results in a higher concentration of consumable material, and less waste.

Cultivating your own cannabis as a home grower is rewarding. It does not take up a lot of time if done on a small scale, and it frees you from participation in much of the cannabis economy. By putting your time, care, energy, attention, and intention into growing a few plants, you'll develop an open energetic rapport with this extraordinary ally.

COMPLEMENTARY HERBS

Other herbs can support your yoga and cannabis in wonderful ways, especially when it comes to enhancing energy and focus. Over the past few decades I have worked with a great many botanicals and have selected the five I consider of the highest value. These are ashwagandha, rhodiola, maca, schisandra, and ginseng. Additionally a healthy lifestyle may include regular consumption of many herbs of great value such as garlic, ginger, turmeric, and various other spices, which impart health benefits of all kinds. But for the purposes of enhancing yoga in some meaningful way along with an infusion of cannabis, these five are my top picks. I have employed each one extensively and have researched each one in the field. Becoming familiar with them has led me to India, China, and Peru. These are botanicals for which I have developed a great understanding of their capacity to impart energy, endurance, stamina, greater alertness and focus, overall vitality, and a sense of well-being.

Ashwagandha, *Withania somnifera*

Of the approximately 7,500 medicinal plants used in India's several-millennia-old tradition of Ayurveda, ashwagandha, *Withania somnifera,* is the most highly prized. Use of the root and its preparations can be traced back as far as four thousand years. Ashwagandha is classified as a *rasayan,* a rejuvenating or life-extending agent. The rasayan are the most esteemed of Ayurveda's herbs, as they imbue the user with life itself. Ashwaganda root appears in remedies for cough, rheumatism, gynecological disorders, fatigue, emaciation, inflammation, ulcers, sore eyes, and diminished brain function.

Ashwagandha is clinically proven to enhance energy, strength, recovery after exertion, sexual function, mental function, and mood. It significantly reduces stress and helps you to get a good night's sleep. It is used equally by men and women and is widely prescribed by physicians to adults with low libido and to improve sexual function. In the system of Ayurvedic medicine, ashwagandha is widely known as the king of the herbs.

Rhodiola rosea

One of the great botanicals available today, *Rhodiola rosea* originates from both Siberia and the Tian Shan mountain range of northwestern China. A well-studied adaptogen, rhodiola defends the body overall and protects general health and well-being. Its anti-stress and fatigue-fighting properties make it one of the most popular botanicals in all of Siberia. And its promotion of energy, endurance, and stamina makes *Rhodiola rosea* a valuable aid for athletes. A small green plant with a golden blossom, rhodiola's beneficial properties lie in the root. Extracts from the roots of the plant have been used by Eastern Bloc athletes for decades to improve overall performance. The root has also enjoyed a very long history for promoting sexual vigor and prowess.

Rhodiola rosea root contains a group of novel compounds that have not been found in other plants. These include rosin, rosavin, and rosarin, known collectively as rosavins. Each of these has been studied, and each appears to make a significant contribution to the plant's unrivaled anti-stress properties. Rhodiola also contains the agent salidroside and protective antioxidants that inhibit the cellular deterioration process of oxidation, which is akin to rusting. Rhodiola also proves to be one of the most effective antidepressive herbs known.

Maca, *Lepidium meyenii*

Maca is an annual plant in the mustard family, which grows in the highlands of Peru and Bolivia and is consumed extensively by the people of that Andean region. Maca is one of only two food crops (the other is potato) that grow at high altitudes in the Junin plateau, which ranges from ten to fifteen thousand feet above sea level. The root of the plant, which resembles a turnip, is harvested and dried. The root is then used in a porridge called mazzamora, and in cookies, baked goods, syrups, juices, blender drinks, and liquors

Maca has been dubbed "Peruvian ginseng," even though it bears no botanical relation to ginseng. But like ginseng, the root is reputed to increase strength, energy, stamina, libido, and sexual function. Since 1998 maca's reputation and popularity has spread throughout Peru and to Europe, Asia, and the United States. Maca is also now vastly popular in China.

Peruvians attribute panacea-like benefits to maca, citing maca as an aphrodisiac and fertility enhancer, a laxative, an aid to rheumatism and respiratory disorders, for stimulating metabolism, regulating hormones, improving memory, combating anemia, and fighting depression.

Schisandra chinensis

Certainly the most super of all super berries, schisandra enjoys a long and distinguished traditional use as a life-extending botanical gem. The berry of schisandra owes its name *wu wei zi* (five-flavored berry) due to its unusual combination of sweet, salty, bitter, pungent, and salty tastes all at once. Schisandra berry is made into various medicinal preparations for longevity and overall vitality.

Schisandra chinensis has enjoyed millennia of use as a general tonic to prolong life, retard the aging process, increase energy, fight fatigue, boost sexual function, enhance physical performance, and promote endurance. Schisandra has significant antioxidant and anti-inflammatory power and is considered one of the most protective of all medicinal plants for general health and specifically for defending and detoxifying the liver. All of the traditional uses of schisandra, with the exception of imparting longer life, have been corroborated in human studies.

Panax ginseng

Ginseng is a tonic herb used for rejuvenation and to reinvigorate the body and mind. It is considered an adaptogen, providing protection against mental, physical, and environmental forms of stress. *Panax ginseng* is a slow maturing perennial herb native to the mountain forests of northeastern China, Korea, and Russia. Ginseng is also cultivated extensively in China, Japan, Korea, Russia, Canada, and Wisconsin in the United States. The roots of ginseng take around five years to mature. Old wild roots are both endangered and highly prized for their purported extra healing powers. Of all medicinal plants *Panax ginseng* is one of the more heavily cultivated on Earth.

The name *panax* derives from Greek and means "panacea" or "cure-all." In Asian medicine dried ginseng root is used as a tonic to revitalize and replenish vital energy, which is referred to as qi or chi. Ginseng is traditionally used as an aid during convalescence and to build immune resistance, reduce susceptibility to illness, and promote vigorous health and longevity. Ginseng extract, ginseng tea, and ginseng liquors are popular throughout Asia. A very large body of science corroborates the traditional uses of ginseng.

✳

I prefer liquid extracts of herbs whenever possible. Ashwagandha, rhodiola, schisandra, and ginseng can all be found in liquid extract form. With these herbs, try taking some right after infusing and before commencing yoga practice. In the case of maca I recommend organic maca root powder. Use this to make a smoothie or some form of blender drink for after practice.

These herbs are excellent companions for both yoga and cannabis. They impart a great many benefits and help to protect against health insults of all types. If you utilize these herbs regularly, you will notice extra energy and improved mental sharpness.

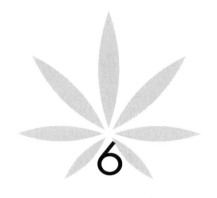

6

PRACTICING
LOTUS AND BUD YOGA

BREATHING

Controlled breathing and specific breathing exercises are key features of a complete yoga program. Breathing is automatic and fundamental to human life. We breathe from the moment we are born, and when we stop breathing, we die. It's very simple. We humans are highly versatile and adaptable. We can go for long periods of time without food, and we can go without water for a few days. We can forgo numerous comforts and pleasures. But if you go without breathing for an extended period of time, you will be released from your mortal form. When we breathe we take in a mixture of gasses, most notably oxygen, which we need to feed our cells. Breathing is the most primary of all forms of nourishment. It's the first thing we do after exiting the birth canal, and the last thing we do before going on to whatever it is that happens after living in a body. We breathe to live.

Though breathing is a simple and natural function, it can be adjusted and modified to yield particular results. Breathing fuels the metabolic process and contributes to the production of energy within us, but it can also be used to build, purify, and strengthen the entire human system. Thus virtually every mode of body-mind development, from all systems of yoga to the various martial arts, utilizes methods of breath control. It is said in some yoga scriptures that when you master the breath, you master your destiny. It is certainly true that as you master the breath, you gain voluntary control over involuntary functions of body and mind, including brainwave activity, pulse rate, and blood pressure.

Proper breathing is important to learn so you can get your practice of yoga off to a good start. Please be sure to practice breathing carefully, according to the instructions given here. Sometimes people feel that they should push themselves at the onset, starting out with great intensity, doing more than is recommended. Refrain from overdoing breathing practice. Even simple, basic breathing methods can be extremely powerful. Because breathing is something natural that we do all the time, it may seem that strenuous practice of breathing exercises would be of little consequence. But this is not the case. As you engage in breathing exercises, a number of things start to happen. Your body begins to detoxify, and poisons are expelled from the liver, kidneys, bowels, and skin. Occasionally you may feel a little light-headed during initial practice, due to the greatly increased amount of oxygen going to your brain. If you find yourself feeling light-headed or dizzy, stop and relax. As you practice controlled breathing, you will feel increasingly energetic and strong. This is because controlled breathing supports all other vital physical functions, while also helping to clear and calm the mind.

We will focus here on two primary breathing methods. The first is the "basic" breath, and the second is the long deep breath. While I would otherwise wish to include breath of fire here as well, I believe that this breath is difficult to convey via a book. For our purposes we do not need to learn or focus on breath of fire.

Practice breathing on an empty stomach to avoid nausea and cramping and to allow your body to feel as free and comfortable as possible.

◈ *The Basic Breath*

Sit in a comfortable position, either cross-legged or in a straight chair. Keep your spine erect, so you are sitting as tall and upright as possible. The bones of your spine are resting one on top of the other, like a stack of coins. Your shoulders and chest are relaxed. Place one hand with the palm flat on your abdomen. This is so you can feel what is happening more easily. Once you are familiar with basic breathing, placing your hand on your abdomen will not be necessary.

Inhale lightly through the nose, and as you do, let your abdomen fill and expand outward. **Exhale** through either the nose or mouth, relaxing the breath. Your chest should not move at all. This breath is much like filling a balloon. As you inhale through your nose, your abdomen expands. As you exhale through the nose or mouth, your abdomen collapses. As simple as this sounds, it is very important, so go over it repeatedly. For about two minutes practice easy, gentle breathing, expanding your abdomen as you inhale through the nose, and letting your abdomen collapse as you gently exhale through the nose or mouth.

The basic breath is the regular, relaxed breathing that you should maintain throughout the day. You may find, however, that you have been breathing in a different way, sucking in your abdomen upon inhaling. This is altogether too common, and it takes practice and concentration to retrain yourself to breathe properly.

Please Note

It is important to inhale through your nose whenever possible. Inhaling through the mouth typically results in shallow breathing and can contribute to dizziness and nervousness. Be sure to inhale regularly through the nose. Exhalation may be either through the nose or mouth.

◈ *The Long Deep Breath*

This is similar to the basic breath, except that it is deeper. To practice this breath, place one hand with the palm flat on your abdomen and one at the center of your chest. This hand placement is for learning this breath, not for regular practice.

As you **inhale** draw the breath in through the nose, filling your abdomen as in the normal breath. But this time continue inhaling until your lungs are also full to the top and your chest is expanded.

Then gently **exhale** through either the nose or mouth.

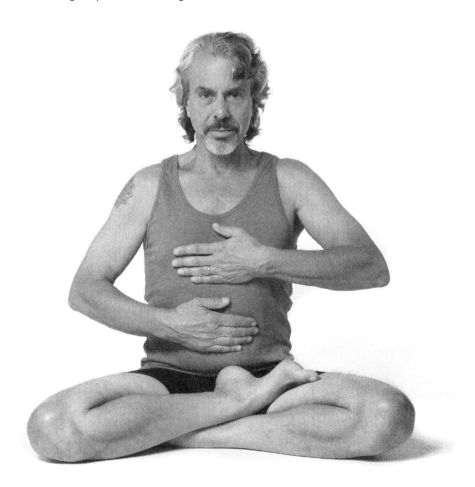

The long deep breath

It is important that you work with this breath until you perform it correctly, easily. The long deep breath is much like filling a glass of water. You pour water in from the top, but the glass fills from the bottom up. It is the same with the breath. Breath comes in from the top of your body but it fills you up from the lower abdomen first, then filling the chest.

Practice this long deep breath for a few minutes every day, until you have perfected it and it comes easily and automatically.

Benefits

Any time you need to relieve stress (except after a large meal, when you may experience discomfort), sit in a relaxed but upright position and breathe long and slowly, drawing the breath deep down inside you and letting it out easily and evenly. Doing this literally washes away tension and will leave you feeling calm, relaxed, and invigorated.

Now that you have practiced breathing, you are ready to begin practicing yoga.

THE POSTURES

Lotus and Bud Yoga

Here we are, at the place that matters most, practice. All ideas, explanations, considerations, and theories are helpful, but only to assist practice.

The methods that follow are all part of True Kundalini yoga, a range of authentic kundalini yoga methods I have accumulated over decades and practiced. These methods have authentic and verifiable histories of traditional practice. You will recognize many of these methods as deriving from classical hatha yoga. This is because hatha yoga is by nature a path to awakening kundalini.

The asanas are arranged in order of practice for maximum effect. While I understand that you may practice what follows in any order you wish, I have sequenced them to naturally follow one another especially to best build energy.

Each of these yoga techniques comes from verifiable tradition, and I have personally practiced each method at least a couple of thousand times. These methods work very well to arouse the kundalini and to open up the energy channels throughout your body and mind.

◇ *Cat Stretch*

Kneel on your hands and knees, with the insteps of your feet flat on the ground. As you **inhale** through the nose, stretch your head as far up and back as you can, while at the same time arching your tailbone up, dropping your spine down. As you **exhale** through the mouth through pursed lips, tuck your chin into your chest, dropping your tailbone and rounding your spine up as high as you can.

Repeat this **40 to 100 times** in a steady rhythm. At the end take a **long deep breath**, hold it for as long as you can comfortably, then **exhale** and relax in a comfortable sitting position.

Benefits

Cat stretch loosens your spine from the base to the top of the neck, while stimulating all the spinal nerves at the same time. This method awakens the entire body and increases circulation to the brain. Loosening and stimulating the spine is an essential first step in any well-designed body-mind energizing regime.

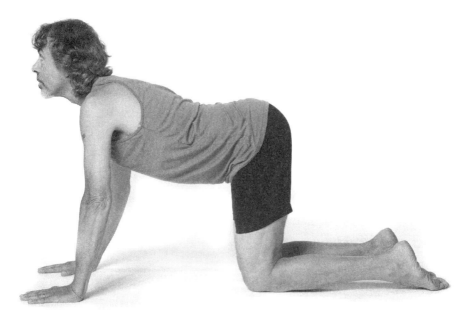

Cat stretch: inhale

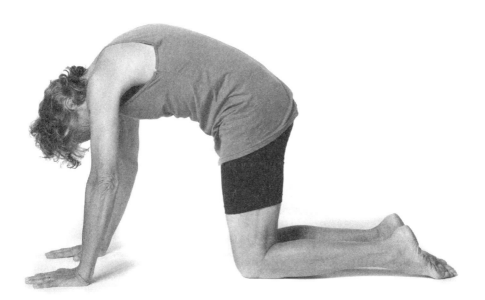

Cat stretch: exhale

◈ *Squat*

Stand with your feet slightly wider than shoulders' width apart. Keeping your feet flat on the ground, bend your knees, lowering your buttocks down between your feet. Your arms rest between your knees. Relax in this position for **a minute or two**. Your breath is normal and at ease.

Squatting may be difficult at first, and you might find it hard to keep your feet flat on the ground without falling backward. If this is the case, you may wish to practice the squat initially by holding on to a table leg or post until you are comfortable in the position.

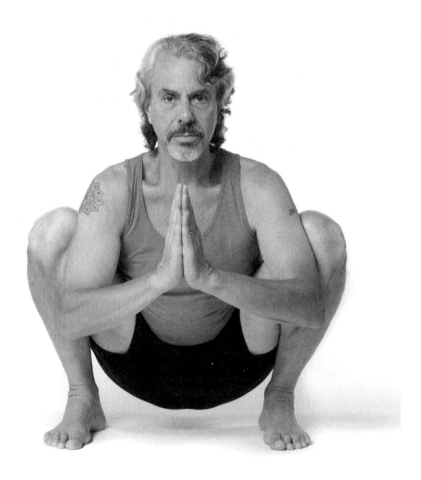

Squat

You will find that gently rocking forward and back in the squat further loosens up the hips, ankles, and spine.

Benefits

Squatting stretches the ligaments in your hips, opens up the pelvis, stretches the lower spine, relieves a sore lower back, strengthens and loosens the ankles, and soothes the entire nervous system. Once you get used to squatting, you'll find that it refreshes tired legs and works tension out of your body very effectively. As you exercise you can return repeatedly to the squat, and it will only do you good. Many people I know take a few squatting breaks of a few minutes' duration during busy work days to refresh themselves. It works.

◈ *Spinal Twist in Easy Pose*

Sit cross-legged, with your spine upright and your hands on your knees. In this position **inhale** moderately through the nose.

As you **exhale** twist and rotate your spine as far as you comfortably can to the left. You can use your hands for leverage to accentuate the motion, but don't force the stretch.

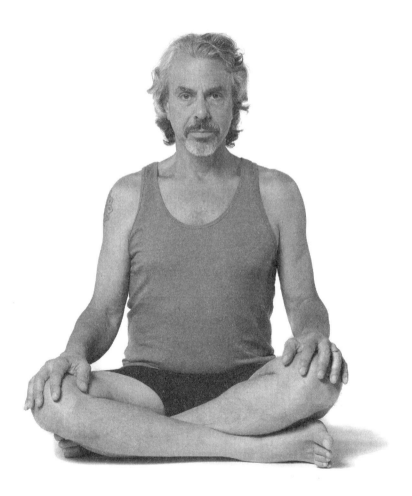

Spinal twist in easy pose, starting position

Inhale lightly as you move back to the center, then **exhale** again, this time as you twist and rotate to the right.

Repeat this motion **20 to 40 times** on both sides, alternately stretching from one side to another in a rhythmic, fluid motion. When you are finished bring yourself back to a centered, upright sitting position, take a **long deep breath**, hold it for as long as you can comfortably, then **exhale** and relax for a moment.

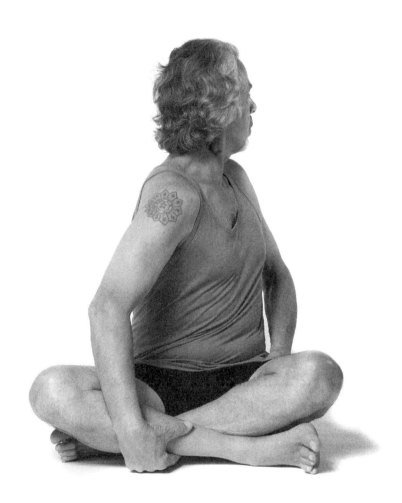

Spinal twist in easy pose to the left

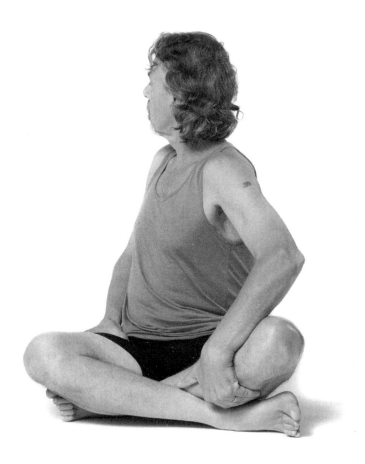

Spinal twist in easy pose to the right

Benefits

Spinal twists further loosen up your spine, increasing the range of spinal rotation. Spinal twists stimulate the lower spine especially, while gently strengthening lower postural muscles. You may hear some "popcorn" in your spine when you practice these twists. That is the sound of vacuums releasing between vertebrae and is nothing to worry about.

◈ Dog Stretch

Start out sitting on the backs of your heels, with the balls of your feet and your knees on the ground. The palms of your hands are flat on the ground right beside your knees. Your arms are straight, your spine is as upright as possible, and your head is up, looking forward.

Inhale, and as you do, straighten your legs, dropping your heels to the ground and raising your buttocks up, and drop your head down with your chin tucked in (see image on page 134).

Exhale, and as you do, bend your legs and bring yourself down to the first position.

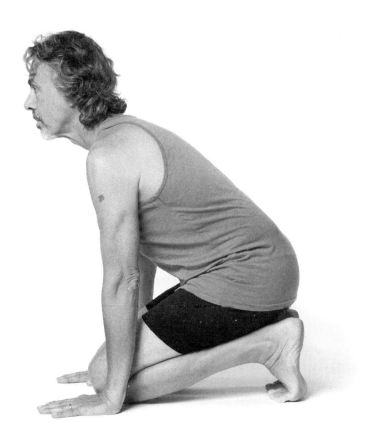

Dog stretch, starting position

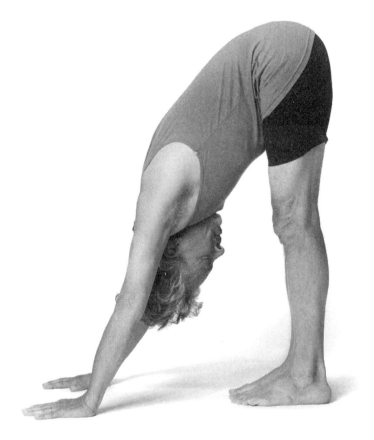

Dog stretch

Repeat dog stretches in a steady rhythm, with strong breathing, **20 to 50 times**.

Benefits

Dog stretches will stretch out, strengthen, and tone your legs. They stretch out the hamstrings and the lower back; loosen the ankles, knees, and hips; strengthen the thighs; increase circulation; and boost metabolism.

◈ *Standing Alternate Leg Stretch*

Stand with your feet half again wider than shoulders' width apart, with your body upright. Your arms are stretched above your head, with your fingers pointing upward and your thumbs interlocked.

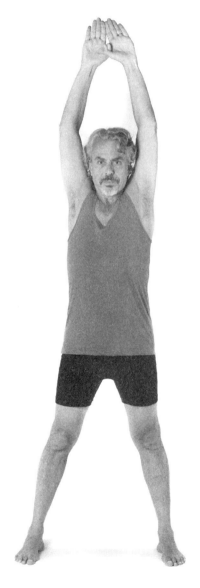

Standing alternate leg stretch,
starting position

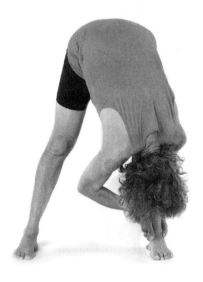
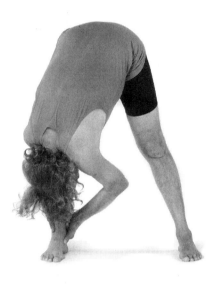

Standing alternate leg stretch
to the left

Standing alternate leg stretch
to the right

Inhale deeply in this upright position, then **exhale**, stretching down over your left leg, touching your head to your knee and flattening your chest against your leg if you can, with your hands clasped behind your ankle.

Inhale back into the fully stretched upright position. Then **exhale**, stretching down over your right leg.

Repeat this stretch **8 to 21 times** on each side, stretching as far down as you can each time. When you have finished come into the upright position, take a long deep breath, and hold the breath for a few seconds. Then exhale and relax.

Benefits

Standing leg stretches open up the nerves and muscles in the backs of the legs, open up the rib cage, and increase respiratory capacity. This method greatly enhances lower spinal flexibility, improves balance, stimulates circulation, and enhances digestion and elimination.

◈ *Standing Triangle Stretch*

Stand with your feet almost twice your shoulders' width apart, with your arms outstretched to the sides, palms down (see image on page 138). **Inhale** in this upright position.

Exhale as you twist, rotate, and turn from the lower waist and hips, bringing your left hand down in front of your right foot, palm flat on the ground. Your right arm is pointing up in the air, and your head is turned up (see image on page 139).

Inhale and lift back into the upright position, and **exhale** down, stretching the same way on the other side.

Repeat the stretch **8 to 21 times** on each side.

Benefits

Standing triangle stretches greatly increase your spinal flexibility, energize spinal nerves, stretch the backs of the legs, strengthen the legs, enhance posture, increase circulation to digestive organs, increase overall circulation, improve balance, enhance intestinal elimination, and increase respiratory capacity.

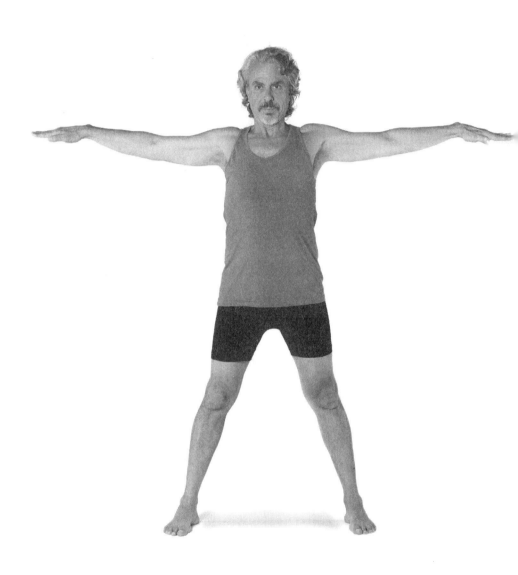

Standing triangle stretch, starting position

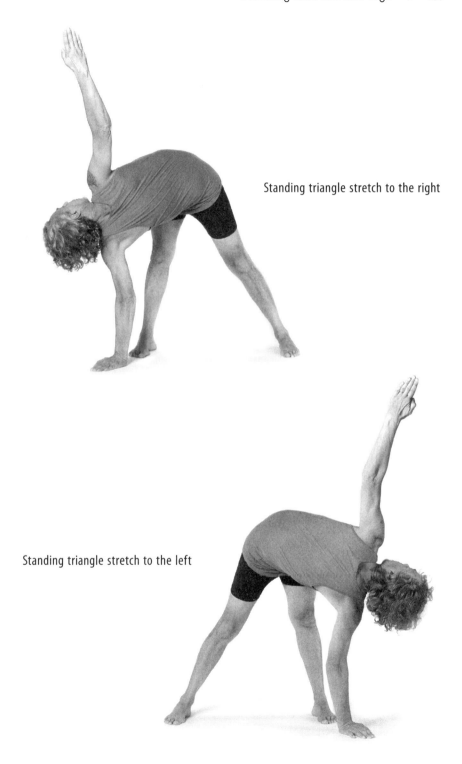

Standing triangle stretch to the right

Standing triangle stretch to the left

◈ *Sitting Head-to-Knee Stretch*

Sit on the ground with your legs extended together in front of you. Your arms are stretching up toward the sky, thumbs locked together. **Inhale** deeply in this position.

Exhale, and as you do, stretch all the way forward, bending from your hips. Ideally, stretch down so that your head rests on your knees and you can catch your feet with your hands. Hold this position for a couple of seconds.

Then **inhale**, and as you do, stretch up into the first position, arms extended up as high as you can.

Repeat sitting head-to-knee stretches in a steady, even rhythm **11 to 21 times**, inhaling up and exhaling down, stretching a little bit further with each breath. When you are finished come up into the upright position, take a **long deep breath**, and hold it for a few seconds. Then **exhale** gently and relax.

Benefits

Sitting head-to-knee stretches open up the backs of your legs, hips, and lower back; strengthen the lower back; strengthen and stretch the spine, torso, and shoulders; and increase circulation and respiratory capacity.

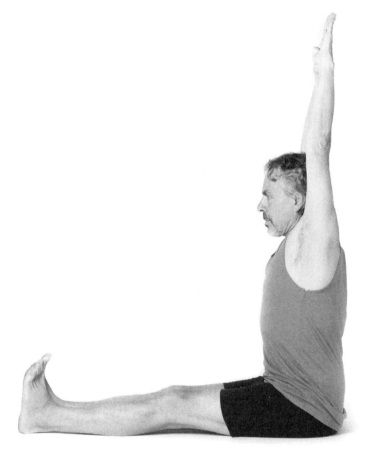

Head-to-knee stretch, starting position

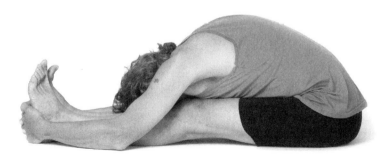

Head-to-knee stretch

◈ *Supine Spinal Twist*

Lie on your back with your legs together, your feet pointing straight upward, and your arms extended straight out to the sides perpendicular to your body with the palms down. **Inhale** in this position.

Exhale, and as you do, stretch your legs over to the left side, bringing your toes down near your left hand. Keep your shoulders and arms firmly planted on the ground as much as possible. The rotation comes from the lower and middle spine.

Inhale back up to the starting upright position.

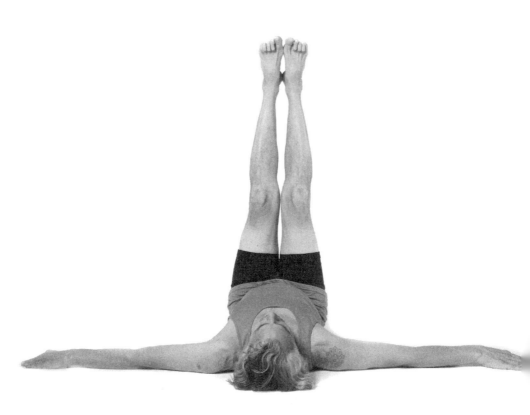

Supine spinal twist, starting position

Repeat the stretch on both sides **7 to 21 times**, with dynamic breathing. When you have finished take a **long deep breath** in the upright position, then **exhale** gently and relax.

Benefits

Supine spinal twists increase your spinal flexibility, strengthen the hips, lower back, and abdomen, and improve digestion and intestinal elimination.

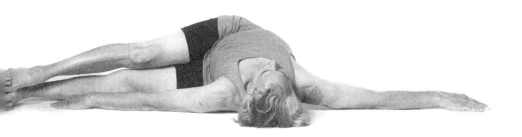

Supine spinal twist to the left

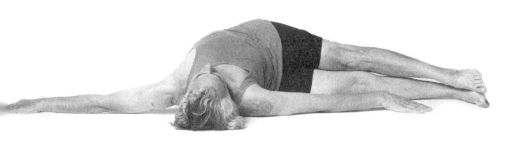

Supine spinal twist to the right

❖ *Chi Kung Double Kick*

Sitting on your tailbone, draw your knees tightly to your chest, with your feet together a few inches off the ground. Your arms are extended in front of you, hands slightly in front of your knees, fingers open.

As you **exhale** evenly through pursed lips, extend your legs straight out, tucking your chin into your chest, clenching your hands into fists, and tucking them close against your armpits. When your legs are fully extended, tense your entire body for a moment.

Inhale as you come back into the first position with your knees drawn up against your chest.

Repeat this exercise **21 to 50 times**, keeping your feet off the ground the whole time. The pace is moderate and smooth.

Benefits

Chi kung double kicks tone and strengthen your abdomen, upper thighs, hips, back, sides, and chest. This is an exceptional exercise that also improves balance and enhances digestion and elimination.

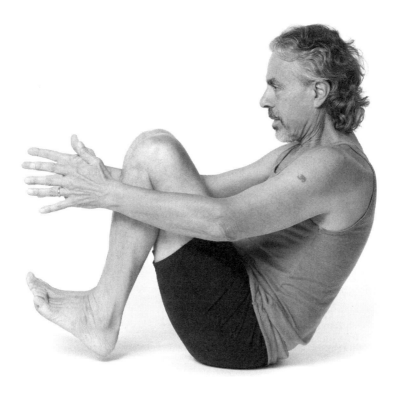

Chi kung double kick, starting position

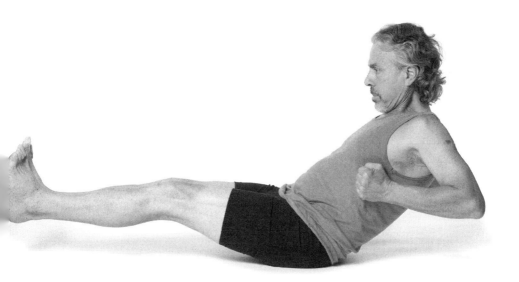

Chi kung double kick, extension

◈ *Chi Kung Turtle Stretch*

Stand in horse stance, with your feet about double your shoulders' width apart. Your feet are parallel to each other; your knees are bent and wide apart. Your back is straight, with a slight inward curve in the lower spine. Your hands are tucked against your mid ribs at the sides, palms up and fingers together.

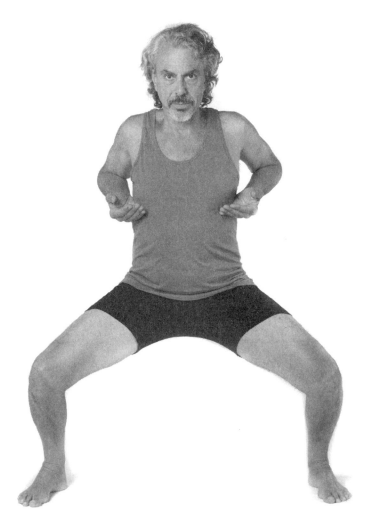

Chi kung turtle stretch, starting position

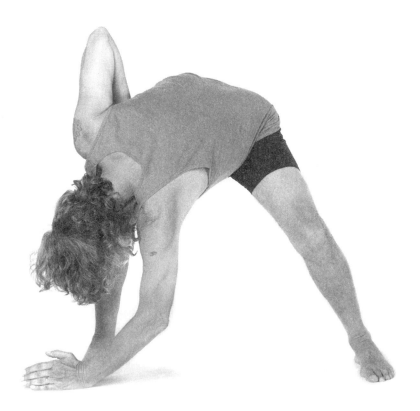

Chi kung turtle stretch to the right

As you **exhale** forcefully through pursed lips, tuck your chin into your chest, bend down, and rotate your trunk to your right, placing the outer edge of your left hand on the ground in front of your right foot.

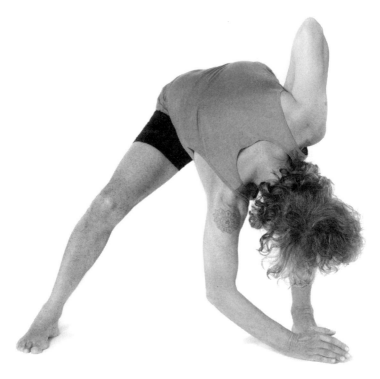

Chi kung turtle stretch to the left

Inhale as you come back up to the starting position. Then **exhale** as you stretch in the same way to your left, and **inhale** up again.

Repeat the turtle stretch **9 to 21 times** on each side.

Benefits

The turtle stretch strengthens your thighs, hips, and lower back, improves posture, and enhances respiration, digestion, and intestinal elimination.

◈ *Chi Kung Fish Stretch*

Start out on your knees and on the balls of your feet, both of which are your shoulders' width apart. You are sitting back on your heels, arms stretched forward with the right hand overlapping the left, and your forehead to the ground (see image on page 150).

Inhale, and as you do, straighten your legs out so that your torso moves forward and up over your arms, which remain perfectly straight, supporting your weight. Keep your chin tucked into your chest. When you are fully extended, your body should be straight as a plank, with arms and legs straight (see image on page 150).

As you **exhale** powerfully through pursed lips, slowly bend your legs, dropping back down to the first position in a steady, controlled manner.

Repeat the chi kung fish stretch **20 to 100 times**, with vigorous breath. Build up to whatever is reasonable for you.

Benefits

Fish stretches strengthen your legs, hips, lower back, shoulders, and arms, increase circulation and balance, and are very stimulating overall. They make your body feel galvanized and strong.

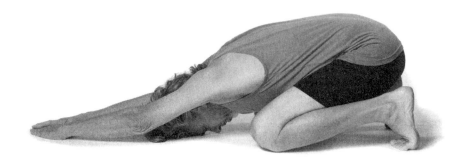

Chi kung fish stretch, starting position

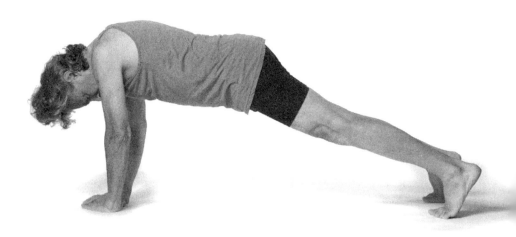

Chi kung fish stretch, extension

◈ *Shakti Breath*

Sit on your knees, buttocks resting on your heels, insteps flat against the ground. Your spine is perfectly straight. Your hands are behind your head, fingers interlocking, with your elbows straight out to the sides.

In this position, **inhale** fully and deeply through the nose, and **hold the breath**.

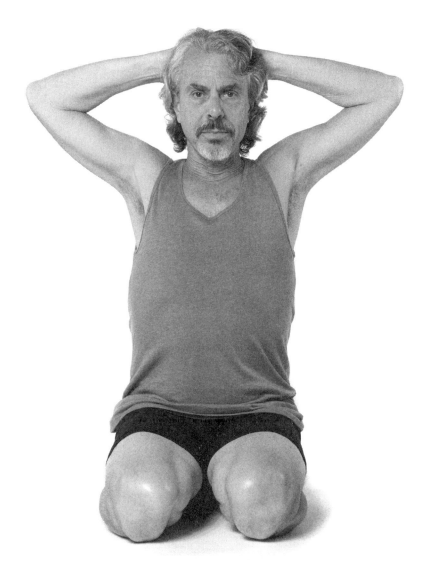

Shakti breath, starting position

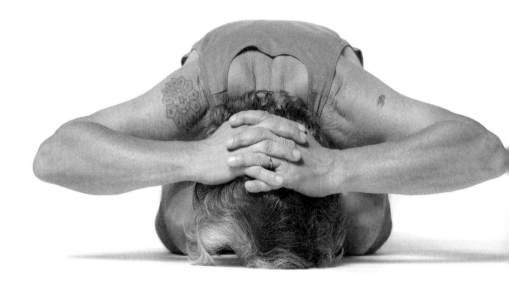

Shakti breath

Holding the breath, bend forward from your hips as far as you can. Ideally your forehead will touch the ground. Your elbows remain straight out to the sides. Hold this downward position to an inner count of seven.

Come back upright to the first position and **exhale** through your mouth forcefully, through pursed lips. This completes one full breath.

Perform this breath **3 to 7 times**. Breathe powerfully, holding the breath firmly, and when you exhale, force the breath out vigorously. After you are finished rest for a moment in a comfortable cross-legged position or in the squat.

Benefits

The shakti breath increases your respiratory capacity, boosts metabolism, strengthens the lower spine, increases circulation to your head, stimulates your brain, and clears your mind. This is an excellent method to perform prior to meditation.

◈ *Initiate's breath*

Stand with your feet approximately shoulders' width apart and your hands on your hips. In this position take a **long deep breath** through the nose and **hold** it.

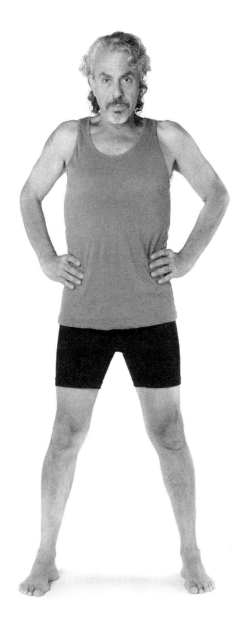

Initiate's breath, starting position

Holding the breath, stretch to your right, and then to the left. Stretch from right to left three times, all the while **holding** in the breath.

Then come upright and exhale forcefully through the mouth through pursed lips. This completes one full breath.

Perform this breath **3 to 7 times**. Breathe powerfully, holding the breath firmly, and when you exhale force the breath out vigorously. After you are finished rest for a moment in a comfortable cross-legged position, or in the squat.

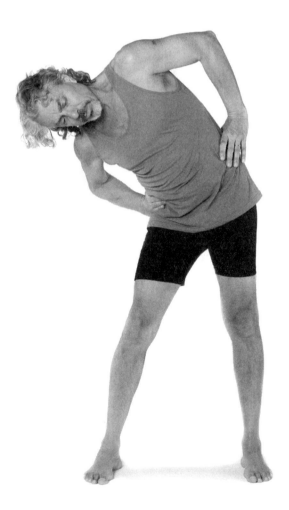

Initiate's breath to the right

Benefits

The initiate's breath increases your respiratory capacity, boosts metabolism, strengthens the lower spine, improves digestion and intestinal elimination, and clears the mind. This also is an excellent practice to perform prior to meditation.

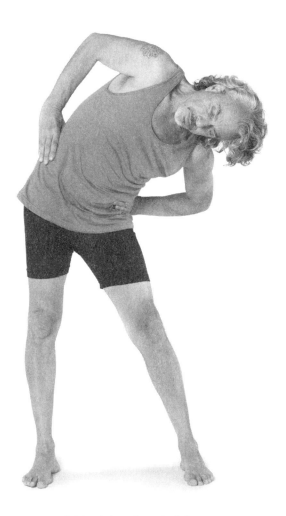

Initiate's breath to the left

MEDITATION

Meditation is beyond thought, beyond our typical experiences of waking, sleeping, and dreaming. At the same time, though, you can meditate while in these states. Meditation is utterly straightforward, yet the process of meditation is also mysterious in terms of what it reveals when we practice. It is immediately available; anyone can sit down and begin to meditate. Yet meditation is also cultivated over a lifetime, like a pearl that accumulates in an oyster from one irritating grain of sand. Meditation exists on the filamentous thin line between negative and positive, between the known and unknown. When you meditate you learn to dwell in pure awareness, consciousness without an object. Initially meditation is a practice, a technique, but over time it becomes a way of living. So meditation is both a method and an all-pervasive way of being.

There are many hundreds of meditation techniques, originating from virtually all spiritual or religious traditions. In their varied forms meditation methods are practiced to clarify the mind, expand awareness, and create inner harmony. There is no ultimate technique of meditation. Instead different practices are temperamentally suited to particular individuals. At the same time most methods will yield benefits for anyone who will invest time and energy in them. Practice is essential with meditation. Meditation is not like a piece of pie. You can't nibble off a little and gain full satisfaction. It takes time and energy and concentration and regular practice to discover the power and value of any valid form of meditation. Casual flirtations with meditation will yield little. Only persistence yields the rewards of meditation practice.

The meditative mind is like a brilliant mirror, which is finely polished and, carrying no images of its own, superbly reflects whatever appears before it. Through meditation you become vividly and brilliantly aware of the present moment. Meditation works very differently from thinking. During thinking the mind is filled with symbols, visual images, words, or other mental products that describe life in some way. But meditation involves dipping into the vast and limitless pool of pure consciousness without abstraction and symbols. The true benefit of meditation practice is a clear, unperturbed mind, a mind that is marvelously aware and attentive, yet unfettered by either stress or limiting concepts.

To derive the most from meditation, make time for daily practice, and do not hurry. No matter how much time you set aside to meditate, let that be a time when you are undisturbed by telephones, conversation, or other external distractions. You will encounter enough internal distractions to keep you well interrupted, fighting for a little bit of clarity. Initially you will find that it is easier to meditate on an empty stomach. This is because after a full meal, blood circulation in the stomach is at an all-time high. At that time, under those conditions, it is often difficult to concentrate and easy to doze off. While you can meditate at any time, it is often easiest to set aside time in the morning upon waking or prior to bed in the evening.

When you meditate wear loose, nonrestrictive clothing, and seat yourself in a comfortable place. Have a blanket on hand as body temperature often drops when meditating. If you can, meditate in a natural setting such as the woods or the beach. Nature has a wonderful way of facilitating meditation, because we come from nature, and we draw physical and spiritual refreshment from being in nature. Wherever you meditate keep that place neat, clean, and attractive. If you can, afford yourself a special spot for meditation only, even if it's just a small corner of a room. Create a special mood by honoring that place.

The following is a seemingly simple yet profoundly valuable method of meditation.

◊ Infused Meditation

Start out by infusing in any manner that works best for you, vaporizing, eating, or smoking. Allow yourself time for the effects of the cannabis to come on, naturally and easily engulfing your senses. Once you are immersed in the expansive high, then seat yourself comfortably in a cross-legged position. Any cross-legged position is fine, provided you keep your spine as erect as possible. You may wish to sit on a small pillow to raise yourself and make it easier to sit erect. Rest your hands on your knees with the palms down; close your eyes; close your mouth gently, resting the tip of your tongue on your upper palate, just behind your front teeth.

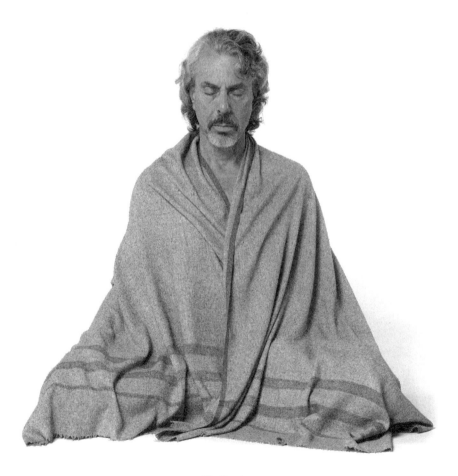

Meditation

In this position breathe steadily and easily through the nose for several minutes. As you do this relax any unnecessary tension in your muscles, except for what you need to sit upright with an erect spine. Let your shoulders, abdomen, and facial muscles be very relaxed. Let your mind settle down as much as possible as you breathe. Throughout this meditation breathing is a key element. It is not necessary to lengthen and deepen the breath greatly, but the breath is slightly deeper than a normal, relaxed breath. Your breath is a steady, even stream, flowing in and out of your body, while your mind gently settles down, becoming more open, spacious, and quiet. Maintain this breathing throughout the entire meditation.

Once you are relaxed and settled, turn your attention to your spine. From the base of the spine to the top of your head, feel the length of your spinal column. This is not visualization, but sensing the energy that is already present, already flowing. As you inhale let the feeling of the breath travel into your body, flowing down your spine to the very base. As you exhale let the feeling of the breath flow up the spine and out the top of your head. As thoughts come and go, neither dwell on them nor fight them. Just keep your attention focused on the full length of your spine and on the sensation of the breath traveling up and down along its length.

Sit this way, focused on the breath and the spine for fifteen minutes or so. Then cease paying attention to your spine, focusing on nothing in particular, just being mindful and expansive. As thoughts arise just let them go. As distractions occur let them go. As the mind squirms and contrives to be noisy, let go of all static and fluctuations. Meditation is conscious non-attachment to any thought or phenomena. To be conscious without thought or disturbance, surrender all thinking and simply dwell in your most essential, peaceful state.

Don't just do something, sit there.
FELIX BLISS

Begin meditation practice for twenty minutes or so, concentrating on the breath and the spine for about fifteen minutes, and remaining in an aware, conscious state without attention on anything for another five minutes or so. As you become increasingly comfortable with practice, meditate for half an hour or more, dividing your time equally between concentrating and breathing into the spine and sitting simply still and alert.

If you practice regularly and consistently, your meditation will deepen. If there is a problem with describing meditation, it is that actually doing so is utterly simple. But our own sense of complexity makes meditation a challenging undertaking. Our minds are busy with thoughts, ideas, notions, memories, fears, projections, and on and on, an endless stream of mental perturbations. It does no good at all to declare to yourself, "I'll stop thinking now," as that is simply more ideation. When thoughts arise allow them to pass by in the parade of chatter that seemingly never ceases. As you do this more and more, that chatter will, in fact, subside.

Benefits

Meditation enables you to tap directly into pure consciousness, the deepest, most refreshing well of being. Meditation practice promotes mental peace and clarity and enhances and vivifies all the senses. Meditation engenders a humbling and inspiring sense of connectedness with all things and fosters innate well-being and happiness. It is a worthy pursuit.

RELAXATION

To live a long, healthy life, one of the essential talents to learn is the art of deep relaxation. To be able to relax deeply upon command is invaluable for shedding stress, relieving fatigue, giving the body and mind profound rest, and refreshing yourself overall.

Having taught relaxation methods in hundreds of classes, I know how hard something as simple as relaxing can actually be. I have watched students fret and fidget and tense and hold themselves in a state of high anxiety, when what they were supposed to be doing is relaxing.

Relaxing, though it is a volitional process, involves letting go, surrendering tension and control. You cannot relax and maintain tight control at the same time. But you can relax voluntarily, maintaining a state of alertness and lucidity while your body seems to slip away.

Deep relaxation involves a measure of trust. You have to be willing to let go of all tension, assured that you will have a friendly experience.

To commence deep relaxation, employ the following method described on pages 162–63.

◇ *Deep Relaxation*

Make sure that you will be warm enough, and that your clothing is loose and nonrestrictive. Put yourself in Savasana, lying flat on your back with your legs fully extended, with your feet about a foot apart. Your arms are also outstretched, with your hands about a foot away from your body, the palms up. Your eyes are closed. In this position begin long, slow breathing for a minute or two. With every exhalation let your body settle more into the ground, as though you are melting into the earth. Let go of any part of your body that is obviously tense.

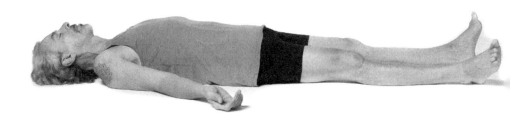

Deep relaxation in Savasana

After a couple of minutes, you are ready to begin more systematic and thorough relaxation. Start by putting your attention at your feet. As you breathe feel your feet as fully as you can. As the breath flows in and out, consciously let go of any tension in your feet. Then move your attention to your lower legs and repeat the process. Breathe slowly and easily, and with every easy breath, let the muscles in your lower legs relax completely. Repeat this process with your knees, your thighs, your pelvis, the lower abdomen, the buttocks and lower back, mid abdomen and mid back, chest and upper back, upper arms, forearms, hands, neck, and face. At every part of your body, take as much time as you need to fully apply your attention to that area. If you are slow and careful and systematic, you will be amazed by how deeply relaxed you can get.

When you have gone through your body, consciously relaxing every part, let your breath become as soft and gentle as possible. Let your attention rest on the breath in a feather-light manner. Do not apply intense concentration; just pay attention in the easiest possible way. At first this may seem hard to do, but with practice you will get the hang of it.

At this point you may drift off to sleep. If you do, there's no harm to it at all. Many people find that going through the progressed relaxation process just described is an excellent prelude to a good night's sleep. Especially if you are a very tense person, relaxing and then passing into sleep may be exactly what you need to do in your initial practice of total relaxation.

If you can put yourself into a profoundly deep, relaxed state with your mind alert, then sooner or later you will make the startling discovery that your body is actually completely asleep, but you are awake. I initially discovered this in a comical way, because I occasionally snore lightly when I sleep on my back. The first time I slept with my mind awake, I thought it was the funniest thing in the world to lie there and listen to my body's light, snoozing snores.

Benefits

It may take you months to become adept at conscious, deep relaxation. But if you will apply yourself to this practice daily, you will find that you can put your body in a totally stress-free, tension-free condition, with your mind in a relaxed, quiescent state, and rouse in ten or twenty minutes, feeling deeply rested and refreshed. Practice is the key. If you put in the time to train yourself to relax deeply, you will be able to rest and refresh yourself in a variety of circumstances. Knowing how to relax deeply is a wonderful, self-empowering talent that will serve you for life.

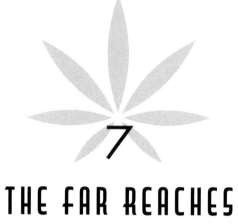

7

THE FAR REACHES

THE MORNING IS BASICALLY ROUTINE. Up before sunrise, shower, coffee overlooking the dawn, yoga, breakfast, time in the water; a few hours of slow and easy entrance into a long and leisurely Caribbean day. My wife, Zoe, and I have a patio ideal for yoga, overlooking the sea. The sky is blue, the air is fresh, nearby hibiscus are blooming madly all around, and a large dog named Daisy is lazing nearby on a chaise longue. She is gigantic, a supersized Rhodesian Ridgeback, all muscle, with a monstrous head and prolific drool. You could put a saddle on this dog. The moment we stepped on the property a week ago, Daisy adopted us as her people. I order sides of bacon for her at breakfast and she, in turn, will eat any intruders. She sleeps near our bed at the front of the cabana and won't even let the night watchman near, though she is fine with the woman who cleans.

I am loose and tanned from leisurely hours of play in the warm silken waters of the Caribbean. The fine beach sand feels just right on long fast walks along the coast. You can go for miles and we do. There is plenty of fresh tropical fruit, there are smoothie bars everywhere, and ganja is prolific. It wafts from behind fences, out of windows and doors, from cars passing by, from restaurants and cafes. The local ganja is abundant, of wonderful quality, and inexpensive. Much of it has a reddish color, and it is all redolent with aromatic terpenes. We have visited a couple of growers nearby to see how they cultivate. Various edible preparations made from the local ganja appear at stands, cafes, and juice bars and vary from gummies to pies to vegan fruit and nut cookies.

The coconut ganja cookie I hold in my hand on the patio smells delectable, made with love and care in a local home kitchen. It came from a woman just down the road. Zoe and I had been roaming around and we came upon a small stand where the woman sold various edibles. She had a hibiscus behind one ear and a small boy, about three years old, with a shy smile. I squatted down and held up my hand for a high five and he smacked my palm like a pro. We all laughed. The woman told me with a smile that the cookie was "Very good choice. You will see." The appearance, fragrance, and overall appeal are just right. As I bite in, hints of nutmeg, cinnamon, and vanilla back the coconut. The cookie is moist from the coconut and an apparent ganja coconut oil. The flavor of the local cannabis adds to a rich sensory experience. You could easily eat way too many of these. That would be an error.

About twenty minutes after eating the cookie, chased with organic coffee, I lie down on the other chaise longue to settle in for an excursion. I have planned this. Daisy raises her immense head and looks me over sleepily, drooling. She appears satisfied. Whatever may take place around me, this place is as secure as a Norman keep. Daisy will protect me, and Zoe remains alert as well. I lie in the warm sun, drifting in the way that happens when the heat and the breeze and the sweet air mingle and work on the body and mind.

As the cookie takes effect, I let go of my tether. I am lying on my back flat in Savasana, arms loose by my sides, palms up. Surrender is key, releasing control and merging into the great current that runs through the all and the everything. My breath settles, muscles loosen, heart rate slows, blood pressure eases, brainwaves harmonize and settle down. The cookie imparts an elevating effect, and I feel a sense of acceleration, a heightening of all sense and sensation.

Elevator in the brain hotel.

DONOVAN, *EPISTLE TO DIPPY*

I offer no resistance. All my energy is in a power surge. The boundaries of my skin vaporize, and I spread out in all directions, bright with light, every atom of my being humming with brilliance. My body is filled with the *nada,* the universal sound current. It is buzzing, chirping, ringing, whining. I focus in on the ringing, and it amplifies as other sounds diminish. I follow the ringing, chasing it across my inner audio landscape.

I feel a great pressure at the very base of my spine. There is a fullness at my perineum, as though something is opening there. As the pressure increases, the ringing of the nada greatly amplifies. Slowly and steadily the pressure rises, incrementally filling my spine from the base on up. It is as though a thick, electrified wand is forcing its way up through my spinal canal. Sounds amplify, the buzzing and ringing joined by clanking, the sounds of birds and insects, a furious rush of water, all together, all louder as the pressure rises. I focus attention simultaneously on the ringing and on the sensation of ever-rising spinal pressure.

I see the force moving up my spine as a serpent, glistening brown, slithering upward toward the top of my head. The pressure is almost too much; the force in my spine strains me. I take in deep breaths, somewhat soothing the intensity. When the pressure reaches the top of my head, it increases, making my crown throb hard. Crackling electricity and loud sounds and overwhelming sensation surge all at once, and then there is this extreme cracking of the bones of my head, breaking apart as the serpent bursts through the top. It is a gleaming-eyed cobra, rising, exultant, spreading its hood. The cobra raises its head up and back, and then in a flash strikes right in the center of my forehead, sinking its fangs deep into my third eye. The piercing sensation and the energy of the action provoke an energetic concussion that blows me apart.

Now there is very little left of me, so little sense of "I," so little story, so little other than oceanic light, bliss, and extreme, ringing energy. The ringing sound is as loud as a train. My entire spine is illuminated with brilliant light and sparkling colors. The kundalini energy rules. I let go more, dissolving, disappearing into ecstatic light. In this hyper-energized, full-throttle state of brilliance, I dwell immersed in bliss. How long this lasts I have no idea, but it seems like a long time. Every cell of my being is cleansed, refreshed, vivified. I feel my heart pumping rich red blood, feel my lungs taking in pure, sweet air. Life current streams through every energetic channel in my body. My mind is burnished and clear. All around me is radiance. My aura is as big as the neighborhood.

After a time I hear a shuffling and some sniffing near me. It takes a few moments, but eventually I turn to see Daisy resting her humongous head inches away on the edge of my chaise longue, observing me up close through big concerned dog eyes as if to inquire if I am all right. I am way past all right, soaked and saturated with light and love and a profound sense of interconnectedness with all things. I reach out and scratch Daisy roughly behind one ear and then the other. She slobbers a little, concern allayed, and settles on the ground with a groan.

The effects of the kundalini awakening last all day and into the night. The next day I still feel brilliant, imbued with massive life force, ready for anything. I am inspired, refreshed, happy, and alive. All this is possible. This is the lotus and the bud, the fusion of yoga and cannabis.

BIBLIOGRAPHY

Avalon, Arthur (Sir John Woodroffe). *The Serpent Power.* New York: Dover Publications, 1928.

Babaji's Devotees, ed. *Babaji Mahavatar the Descent of Eternity Into Time.* Amsterdam: Shri Hairakhan Baba Prachar Sangh Foundation, 1983.

———. *Hariakhan Baba, Known, Unknown.* Davis, Calif.: Sri Rama Foundation, 1975.

Bennett, Chris. *Cannabis and the Soma Solution.* Walterville, Ore.: TrineDay LLC, 2010.

Brahmachari, Dhirendra. *Yogic Suksma Vyayama.* Delhi: Dhirendra Yoga Publications, 1973.

Briggs, George Weston. *Gorakhnath and the Kanphata Yogis.* Delhi: Shri Jainendra Press, 1982.

Brown, David T., ed. *Cannabis: The Genus Cannabis.* Reading, UK: Harwood Academic Publishers, 1978.

Burton, Sir Richard Francis, trans. *The Book of the Thousand Nights and a Night.* London: The Burton Club, 1885.

Cherniak, Lawrence. *The Great Books of Hashish.* 3 vols. Berkeley: And Or Press, 1979.

Clark, Robert C., and Mark D. Merlin. *Cannabis Evolution and Ethnobotany.* Berkeley: University of California Press, 2013.

Clarke, Robert Connell. *Hashish!.* Los Angeles: Red Eye Press, 1998.

Coakley, T. W. *Keef: A Story of Intoxication, Love & Death.* Port Townsend, Wash.: Process Media, 2017.

Cooke, Mordecai. *The Seven Sisters of Sleep.* Rochester, Vt.: Park Street Press, 1997.

Dass, Baba Hari. *The Yellow Book: The Sayings of Baba Hari Dass.* New Mexico: Lama Foundation, 1974.

Dass, Ram. *Be Here Now.* San Cristobal, N.Mex.: Lama Foundation, 1971.

Evans-Wentz, W. Y. *Tibetan Yoga and Secret Doctrines.* New York: Oxford University Press, 1958.

Fremantle, Francesca, and Chogyam Trungpa. *The Tibetan Book of the Dead.* Boulder: Shambhala Publications, 1975.

Germano, Carl. *Road to Ananda.* New York: Healthy Living Publishing, 2018.

Gray, Stephen, and Julie A. Holland. *Cannabis and Spirituality.* Rochester, Vt.: Park Street Press, 2016.

Grotenhermen, Franjo, and Ethan Russo, eds. *Cannabis and Cannabinoids: Pharmacology, Toxicology, and Therapeutic Potential.* New York: The Hayworth Press, 2002.

Hittleman, Richard. *Richard Hittleman's Yoga: 28 Day Exercise Plan.* New York: Workman, 1972.

Jand, K. L. *Immortal Babaji and His Lilas.* Nainital, India: Haidakhanwale Baba's Ashram, 1980.

Kelder, Peter. *The Five Rites of Rejuvenation.* Vista, Calif.: Borderland Sciences Research Foundation, 1975.

Kimmens, Andrew C., ed. *Tales of Hashish.* New York: William Morrow, 1997.

Krishna, Gopi. *Living with Kundalini: The Autobiography of Gopi Krishna.* Boston: Shambhala Publications, 1993.

Krishnamurti, J. *The Only Revolution.* New York: Harper & Row, 1977.

Lawrence, Robyn Griggs. *The Cannabis Kitchen Cookbook.* New York: Skyhorse Publishing, 2015.

———. *Pot in Pans: A History of Eating Cannabis.* Lanham, Md.: Rowman & Littlefield, 2019.

Lee, Martin A. *Smoke Signals.* New York: Scribner, 2012.

Lewin, Lewis. *Phantastica.* Rochester, Vt.: Park Street Press, 1998.

MacCallum, C. A. and E. B. Russo. "Practical considerations in medical cannabis administration and dosing." *European Journal of Internal Medicine* 49 (2018): 12–19.

McPartland, John M., Geoffrey W. Guy, and William Hegman. "Cannabis is indigenous to Europe and cultivation began during the Copper or Bronze age: a probabilistic synthesis of fossil pollen studies." *Vegetation History and Archaeobotany* 27 (2018): 635–48.

Mechoulam, Raphael, ed. *Cannabinoids as Therapeutics.* Basel, Germany: Birkhauser, 2005.

Mishra, Rammurti A. *Fundamentals of Yoga.* New York: The Julian Press, 1987.

Prabhavanandaand, Swami, and Christopher Isherwood. *How to Know God: The Yoga Aphorisms of Patanjali.* Hollywood: Vedanta Press, 1953.

Rajneesh, Bhagwan. *The Book of the Secrets.* New York: Osho International, 1975.

Robinson, Rowan. *The Great Book of Hemp.* Rochester, Vt.: Park Street Press, 1996.

Rudrananda, Swami. *Spiritual Cannibalism.* Woodstock, NY: The Overlook Press, 1987.

Sanella, Lee. *The Kundalini Experience.* Lower Lake, Calif.: Integral Publishing, 1987.

Satchidananda, Swami. *Integral Yoga Hatha.* Buckingham, Va.: Integral Yoga Publications, 1995.

Schultes, Richard Evans, and Albert Hofmann. *Plants of the Gods.* New York: Alfred Van Der Marck, 1979.

Sinh, Panchan, trans. *The Hatha Yoga Pradipika.* Delhi: Oriental Books Reprint Corporation, 1980.

Sivananda, Swami. *Kundalini Yoga.* Garhwal Himalayas, India: The Divine Life Society, 1980.

Toklas, Alice B. *The Alice B. Toklas Cook Book.* New York: Harper & Brothers, 1954.

Vasu, Rai Bahadur Chandra. *The Siva Samhita.* Delhi: Oriental Books Reprint Corporation, 1979.

Vishnudevananda, Swami. *The Complete Illustrated Book of Yoga.* New York: The Julian Press, 1960.

Vivekananda, Swami. *Raja Yoga*. New York: Ramakrishna-Vivekananda Center, 1995.

Von Bibra, Baron Ernst. *Plant Intoxicants*. Rochester, Vt.: Healing Arts Press, 1995.

Yogananda, Paramahansa. *Autobiography of a Yogi*. Los Angeles: Self-Realization Fellowship, 1974.

INDEX